Super Easy Anti-Inflammatory Diet Cookbook for Beginners

2000 Days of Healthy & Delicious Recipes with Simple Ingredients and a 30-Day Meal Plan to Reduce Inflammation, Boost Your Immune System, and Detox Your Body

Enjoy Nutritious Meals with Unmatched Flavor

Barry Vesper

TABLE OF CONTENTS

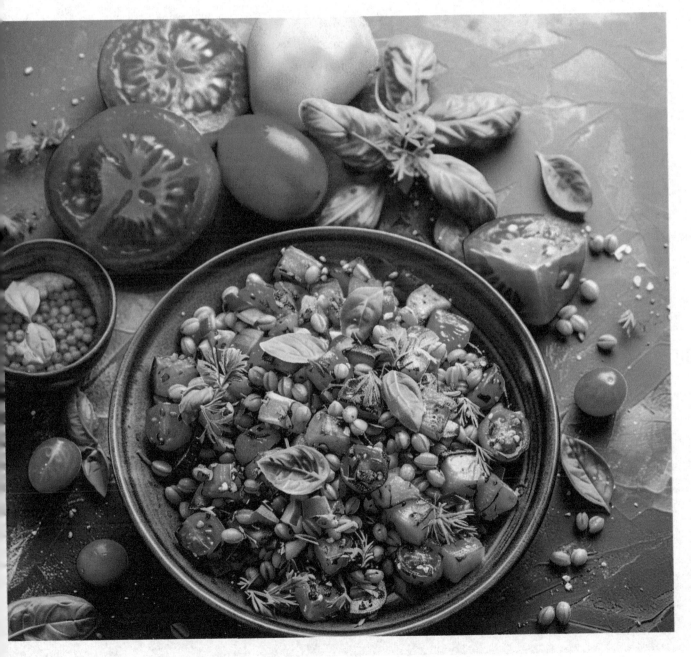

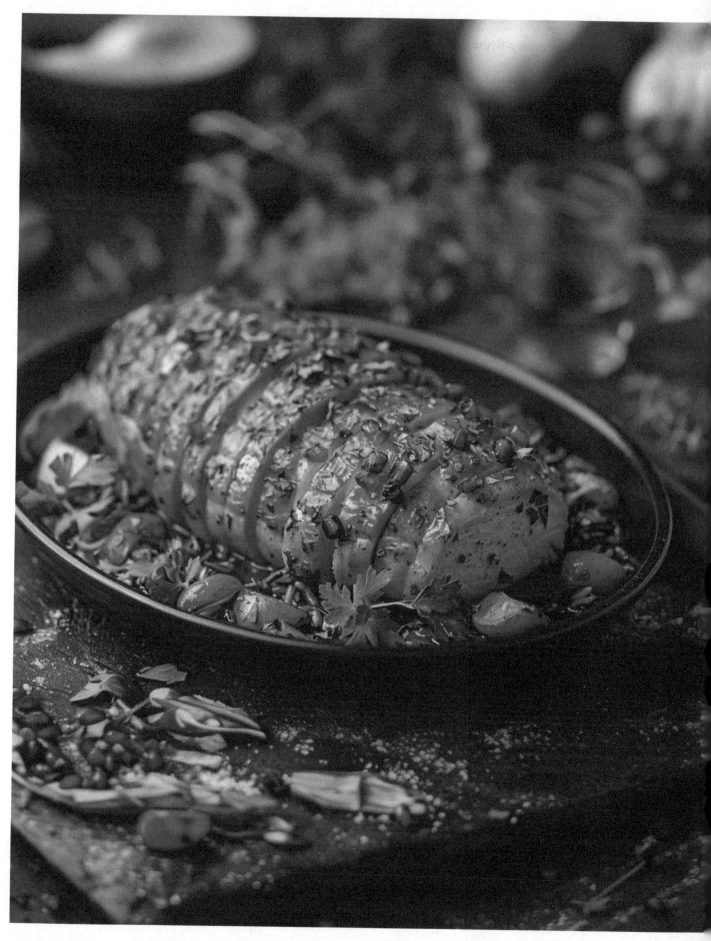

INTRODUCTION

Dear readers,

Barry Vesper, a distinguished chef and expert in anti-inflammatory cooking, shares his culinary wisdom in this comprehensive guide. This book is crafted to help you enjoy the benefits of healthy, delicious meals every day, making it a perfect addition to your wellness journey.

The anti-inflammatory diet offers a wonderful combination of simplicity, versatility, and health benefits. By focusing on nutrient-dense foods and simple ingredients, you can create meals that are both nourishing and flavorful. This diet emphasizes whole foods that reduce inflammation, boost the immune system, and detox the body, making it ideal for everything from hearty breakfasts to satisfying dinners. Cooking with these ingredients requires minimal effort, leading to healthier meals without compromising taste. Its ability to include a variety of foods makes it perfect for family meals and everyday dining.

With Barry Vesper as your guide, your journey to better health through an anti-inflammatory diet will be both straightforward and enjoyable. His expertise and passion will inspire you to create extraordinary meals, turning every meal into a healthful culinary experience. Embrace the limitless possibilities of the anti-inflammatory diet and enjoy the rich flavors and health benefits it brings. Happy cooking!

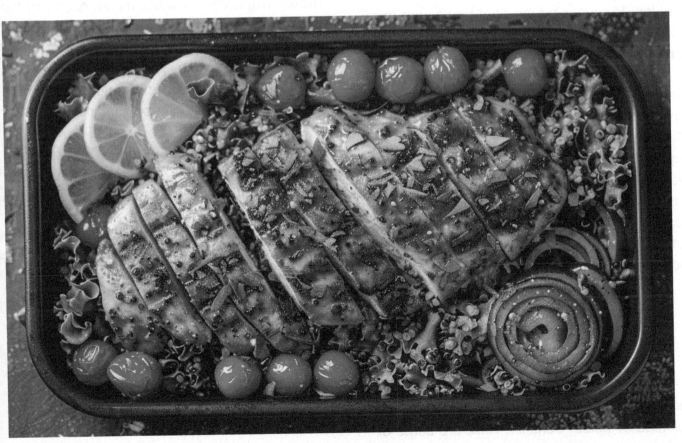

CHAPTER 1: UNDERSTANDING INFLAMMATION

Welcome to Your Anti-Inflammatory Journey

Welcome to "Anti-Inflammatory Diet Cookbook for Beginners" – your essential guide to embracing a healthier, inflammation-free lifestyle. Whether you're a seasoned home cook or just starting to find your way around the kitchen, this book is designed to help you understand the power of food in combating inflammation and improving your overall well-being. Inflammation is a natural response by our body's immune system to fight off infections and heal injuries. However, chronic inflammation can lead to a host of health issues, including arthritis, heart disease, and diabetes. By choosing the right foods, you can reduce chronic inflammation and enjoy a more vibrant, energetic life.

The anti-inflammatory diet focuses on consuming foods that help reduce chronic inflammation. This diet is rich in fruits, vegetables, whole grains, lean proteins, and healthy fats, particularly omega-3 fatty acids found in fish, flaxseeds, and walnuts. These foods are packed with antioxidants, vitamins, and minerals that support the immune system and reduce inflammation.

Benefits of Reducing Inflammation

Reducing inflammation through diet offers a multitude of health benefits. Here are some of the most significant advantages you can expect:

Improved Heart Health: Chronic inflammation is a major risk factor for heart disease. An anti-inflammatory diet can lower cholesterol levels, reduce blood pressure, and improve overall cardiovascular health.

Enhanced Joint Function: For those suffering from arthritis or other joint issues, reducing inflammation can alleviate pain and improve mobility. Foods rich in antioxidants and omega-3 fatty acids can be particularly beneficial.

Better Digestive Health: Inflammation in the gut can lead to conditions like irritable bowel syndrome (IBS) and inflammatory bowel disease (IBD). An anti-inflammatory diet promotes a healthy gut microbiome and reduces symptoms of these conditions.

Stronger Immune System: By reducing chronic inflammation, you can enhance your immune system's ability to fight off infections and illnesses. This leads to fewer colds, flu, and other common ailments.

Weight Management: Inflammation is linked to obesity and metabolic syndrome. An anti-inflammatory diet can help you maintain a healthy weight by improving insulin sensitivity and reducing cravings for unhealthy foods.

Increased Energy Levels: Chronic inflammation can cause fatigue and low energy. By eating anti-inflammatory foods, you can boost your energy levels and feel more vibrant throughout the day.

Mental Clarity and Mood: Inflammation has been linked to mental health issues such as depression and anxiety. An anti-inflammatory diet can support brain health, leading to improved mood and cognitive function.

By adopting an anti-inflammatory diet, you are taking a proactive step towards a healthier, more fulfilling life. This book will guide you through delicious recipes and practical tips to help you enjoy all these benefits and more.

What is Inflammation?

Inflammation is a vital part of the body's immune response. It's the process your body uses to fight off foreign invaders, such as viruses and bacteria, and to heal injuries. When something harmful or irritating affects a part of your body, there is a biological response to try to remove it. This response involves the immune system, blood vessels, and cells. Inflammation can be classified into two types: acute and chronic.

Acute Inflammation

Acute inflammation is the body's immediate response to an injury or infection. It's a short-term process that usually resolves within a few days or weeks. This type of inflammation is characterized by redness, heat, swelling, pain, and loss of function at the site of injury or infection.

Chronic Inflammation

Chronic inflammation, on the other hand, is a long-term condition that can last for months or even years. This prolonged inflammation can lead to tissue damage and contribute to the development of various diseases, including heart disease, diabetes, cancer, and autoimmune disorders.

Chronic inflammation can be subtle, often going unnoticed for years while quietly wreaking havoc on the body. It can result from a variety of factors, including poor diet, lack of exercise, chronic stress, and exposure to environmental toxins. Understanding and addressing the causes of chronic inflammation is crucial for maintaining overall health and preventing disease.

Common Causes of Chronic Inflammation

Poor Diet: Consuming a diet high in processed foods, sugar, trans fats, and refined carbohydrates can contribute to chronic inflammation. These foods can disrupt the balance of good and bad bacteria in the gut, leading to an inflammatory response.

Lack of Physical Activity: Sedentary lifestyles are associated with higher levels of inflammatory markers. Regular exercise helps reduce inflammation by improving circulation, reducing fat tissue, and enhancing the body's immune response.

Stress: Chronic stress can activate inflammatory pathways in the body. The release of stress hormones like cortisol can lead to persistent inflammation, affecting both physical and mental health.

Environmental Toxins: Exposure to pollutants, chemicals, and other environmental toxins can trigger inflammation. These substances can enter the body through the air we breathe, the water we drink, and the products we use, leading to a chronic inflammatory state.

Infections: Persistent infections, whether bacterial, viral, or fungal, can cause chronic inflammation. Conditions like hepatitis, tuberculosis, and certain viral infections are known to provoke long-term inflammatory responses.

Autoimmune Disorders: In autoimmune diseases, the immune system mistakenly attacks healthy tissues, leading to chronic inflammation. Conditions like rheumatoid arthritis, lupus, and multiple sclerosis fall into this category.

Obesity: Excess fat tissue, particularly around the abdomen, produces inflammatory cytokines. This can create a state of low-grade, chronic inflammation that contributes to various metabolic disorders.

How Diet Affects Inflammation

Diet plays a crucial role in either promoting or reducing inflammation in the body. The foods we consume can influence our immune system and inflammatory processes in significant ways. Here's how different dietary choices impact inflammation:

Pro-Inflammatory Foods: Diets high in refined sugars, processed foods, and unhealthy fats (such as trans fats and saturated fats) can trigger inflammatory responses. These foods can increase the levels of inflammatory markers in the blood and disrupt the balance of gut microbiota,

which is essential for maintaining immune health.

Anti-Inflammatory Foods: Foods rich in antioxidants, fiber, and healthy fats help combat inflammation. Fruits and vegetables, especially those high in vitamins C and E, and polyphenols, have anti-inflammatory properties. Whole grains, nuts, seeds, fatty fish (like salmon and mackerel), and olive oil are also beneficial.

Omega-3 vs. Omega-6 Fatty Acids: While omega-6 fatty acids, found in many vegetable oils, can promote inflammation when consumed in excess, omega-3 fatty acids are known for their anti-inflammatory effects. Balancing the intake of these fats is crucial for managing inflammation. Omega-3 fatty acids are found in fatty fish, flaxseeds, chia seeds, and walnuts.

Gut Health: A healthy gut microbiome is essential for regulating inflammation. Consuming probiotics (found in yogurt, kefir, sauerkraut, and other fermented foods) and prebiotics (found in fiber-rich foods like garlic, onions, and bananas) supports a healthy gut flora, which in turn helps reduce inflammation.

Spices and Herbs: Certain spices and herbs, such as turmeric, ginger, and garlic, have potent anti-inflammatory properties. Incorporating these into your diet can help manage and reduce inflammation naturally.

This book provides you with recipes and tips to help you incorporate more anti-inflammatory foods into your daily meals, paving the way for a healthier, more vibrant life.

Essential Foods For Anti-inflammatory Diet

Fruits and Vegetables

Fruits and vegetables are the cornerstone of an anti-inflammatory diet. They are rich in antioxidants, vitamins, minerals, and fiber, all of which help combat inflammation and support overall health.

Berries: Blueberries, strawberries, raspberries, and blackberries are packed with antioxidants and phytochemicals that reduce inflammation and oxidative stress.

Leafy Greens: Spinach, kale, Swiss chard, and collard greens are high in vitamins A, C, and K, as well as anti-inflammatory compounds like flavonoids.

Cruciferous Vegetables: Broccoli, cauliflower, Brussels sprouts, and cabbage contain sulforaphane, a powerful anti-inflammatory compound.

Tomatoes: Rich in lycopene, tomatoes help reduce inflammation and lower the risk of chronic diseases.

Citrus Fruits: Oranges, lemons, limes, and grapefruits are high in vitamin C, which is essential for immune function and inflammation control.

Root Vegetables: Sweet potatoes, carrots, and beets are excellent sources of beta-carotene and other antioxidants.

Whole Grains and Legumes

Whole grains and legumes are vital for an anti-inflammatory diet due to their high fiber content and abundance of nutrients. They help regulate blood sugar levels and provide sustained energy.

Whole Grains: Brown rice, quinoa, oats, barley, and whole wheat are rich in fiber, vitamins, and minerals. These grains help reduce inflammation and improve gut health.

Legumes: Beans, lentils, chickpeas, and peas are excellent sources of protein, fiber, and essential nutrients. They are low in fat and help stabilize blood sugar levels, reducing inflammation.

Buckwheat and Millet: These gluten-free grains are high in fiber and antioxidants, making them great additions to an anti-inflammatory diet.

Healthy Fats and Oils

Healthy fats are crucial for reducing inflammation and promoting heart health. Focus on incorporating unsaturated fats and omega-3 fatty acids into your diet.

Olive Oil: Extra-virgin olive oil is rich in monounsaturated fats and antioxidants. It has strong anti-inflammatory properties and is a staple of the Mediterranean diet.

Avocados: Packed with monounsaturated fats, fiber, and phytochemicals, avocados help reduce inflammation and improve heart health.

Nuts and Seeds: Almonds, walnuts, flaxseeds, chia seeds, and hemp seeds are excellent sources of omega-3 fatty acids, fiber, and antioxidants.

Fatty Fish: Salmon, mackerel, sardines, and trout are high in omega-3 fatty acids, which are known to reduce inflammation and support brain and heart health.

Coconut Oil: While coconut oil contains saturated fats, it also has anti-inflammatory properties and can be used in moderation as part of a balanced diet.

Herbs and Spices

Herbs and spices not only add flavor to your meals but also contain potent anti-inflammatory compounds.

Turmeric: Curcumin, the active ingredient in turmeric, has powerful anti-inflammatory and antioxidant properties. It's especially effective when paired with black pepper, which enhances its absorption.

Ginger: Ginger contains gingerol, a compound with strong anti-inflammatory and antioxidant effects. It can help reduce muscle pain and soreness.

Garlic: Rich in sulfur compounds, garlic has anti-inflammatory and immune-boosting properties.

Cinnamon: Cinnamon helps regulate blood sugar levels and has anti-inflammatory benefits.

Rosemary and Thyme: These herbs are rich in antioxidants and can help reduce inflammation.

Protein Sources

Protein is essential for building and repairing tissues, and certain protein sources can help reduce inflammation.

Fatty Fish: As mentioned, fatty fish like salmon, mackerel, and sardines are excellent sources of anti-inflammatory omega-3 fatty acids.

Lean Poultry: Chicken and turkey are good sources of lean protein without the inflammatory effects of red meat.

Plant-Based Proteins: Tofu, tempeh, edamame, and other soy products provide high-quality protein and are excellent for reducing inflammation.

Eggs: Eggs are a good source of protein and nutrients. Opt for pasture-raised eggs, which are higher in omega-3 fatty acids.

Nuts and Seeds: In addition to being healthy fats, nuts and seeds also provide plant-based protein.

Common Myths About Anti-Inflammatory Diet

Myth 1: An Anti-Inflammatory Diet is Too Restrictive: Many people believe that following an anti-inflammatory diet means giving up all their favorite foods. In reality, this diet is about making healthier choices and incorporating a wide variety of delicious, nutrient-dense foods. You can still enjoy many of your favorite meals with a few adjustments to make them anti-inflammatory.

Myth 2: All Fats are Bad: Not all fats contribute to inflammation. In fact, healthy fats like those found in olive oil, avocados, nuts, and fatty fish are essential for reducing inflammation and supporting overall health. The key is to avoid trans fats and limit saturated fats.

Myth 3: Anti-Inflammatory Foods are Expensive: While some anti-inflammatory foods can be costly, there are plenty of affordable options. Fresh fruits, vegetables, whole grains, legumes, and some healthy fats are budget-friendly and can be easily incorporated into your meals.

Myth 4: You Have to Give Up All Animal Products: While plant-based foods are emphasized in an anti-inflammatory diet, you don't have to become a vegetarian or vegan. Lean proteins like fish, poultry, and eggs can be included in moderation.

Myth 5: Anti-Inflammatory Diet is Only for Those with Chronic Illnesses: While this diet is beneficial for managing chronic inflammation and related illnesses, it's also a great choice for anyone looking to improve their overall health. Reducing inflammation can lead to better energy levels, improved mood, and a lower risk of various diseases.

How to Adjust Recipes for Allergies

Dairy Allergies: Replace dairy products with plant-based alternatives like almond milk, coconut milk, or oat milk. Nutritional yeast can be used as a cheese substitute for a similar flavor.

Gluten Allergies: Opt for gluten-free grains like quinoa, rice, buckwheat, and millet. Use gluten-free flours such as almond flour, coconut flour, and gluten-free oat flour for baking and cooking.

Nut Allergies: Substitute nuts with seeds like sunflower seeds, pumpkin seeds, and hemp seeds. Use seed butters, such as sunflower seed butter, as a replacement for nut butters.

Egg Allergies: Use flaxseeds or chia seeds as an egg substitute in baking. Mix 1 tablespoon of ground flaxseeds or chia seeds with 3 tablespoons of water and let it sit for a few minutes to create a gel-like consistency.

Soy Allergies: Replace soy products with alternatives like coconut aminos (for soy sauce), and use legumes, nuts, and seeds for protein instead of tofu or tempeh.

Lifestyle Tips For Reducing Inflammation

1. Importance of Regular Exercise

Cardiovascular Exercise: Activities like walking, running, swimming, and cycling boost heart health and help reduce inflammation. Aim for at least 150 minutes of moderate aerobic activity or 75 minutes of vigorous activity per week.

Strength Training: Building muscle through resistance exercises like weight lifting or bodyweight workouts can help reduce inflammatory markers. Try to incorporate strength training exercises at least two days a week.

Flexibility and Balance: Practices such as yoga, Pilates, and stretching improve flexibility and balance, reduce stress, and can lower inflammation levels. These activities also promote relaxation and mental well-being.

2. Stress Management Techniques

Deep Breathing: Practicing deep, diaphragmatic breathing can calm the nervous system and reduce stress. Try taking slow, deep breaths in through your nose, holding for a few seconds, and exhaling through your mouth.

Meditation: Regular meditation practice can lower stress levels and reduce inflammation. Even a few minutes of mindfulness meditation each day can make a significant difference.

Exercise: Physical activity is a natural stress reliever. As mentioned earlier, regular exercise helps lower stress hormones and promotes the release of endorphins, which improve mood.

Hobbies: Engaging in hobbies and activities you enjoy can be a great way to relieve stress. Whether it's reading, gardening, painting, or playing a musical instrument, taking time for yourself is important.

Social Support: Connecting with friends, family, or support groups can provide emotional support and help manage stress. Don't hesitate to reach out to loved ones when you're feeling overwhelmed.

3. Quality Sleep and Its Role in Health

Establish a Routine: Try to go to bed and wake up at the same time every day, even on weekends.

Create a Sleep-Friendly Environment: Make your bedroom a comfortable and relaxing space. Keep it cool, dark, and quiet, and invest in a good mattress and pillows.

Limit Screen Time: Reduce exposure screens at least an hour before bedtime.

Avoid Stimulants: Limit caffeine and nicotine intake, especially in the hours leading up bedtime. These substances can disrupt sleep patterns.

Relaxation Techniques: Engage in relaxing activities before bed, such as reading, listening to calming music, or taking a warm bath. These can help signal to your body that it time to wind down.

4. Hydration and Its Benefits

Drink Plenty of Water: Aim to drink at least eight 8-ounce glasses of water a day, or more if you are physically active or live in a hot climate. Carry a reusable water bottle with you to make it easier to stay hydrated throughout the day.

Hydrating Foods: Incorporate water-rich foods into your diet, such as cucumbers, watermelon, oranges, and strawberries. These not only provide hydration but also essential vitamins and minerals.

Limit Dehydrating Beverages: Reduce your intake of alcohol and caffeinated drinks, as they can lead to dehydration. If you do consume these beverages, be sure to balance them with plenty of water.

Monitor Hydration Levels: Pay attention to your body's signals, such as thirst and the color of your urine. Light yellow urine typically indicates proper hydration, while darker urine may signal a need for more water.

5. Mindfulness and Relaxation Practices

Mindfulness Meditation: Practicing mindfulness involves focusing on the present moment without judgment. It can reduce stress and inflammation by promoting relaxation and mental clarity. Try setting aside a few minutes each day to practice mindfulness meditation.

Yoga: Yoga combines physical postures, breathing exercises, and meditation to promote relaxation and reduce stress. It can help lower inflammatory markers and improve overall health.

Progressive Muscle Relaxation: This technique involves tensing and then slowly relaxing each muscle group in the body, promoting physical relaxation and reducing stress.

Guided Imagery: Guided imagery involves visualizing calming and peaceful scenes or experiences. It can help reduce stress and promote relaxation.

Deep Breathing Exercises: Practicing deep breathing exercises can activate the body's relaxation response, reducing stress and inflammation. Try inhaling deeply through your nose, holding for a few seconds, and exhaling slowly through your mouth.

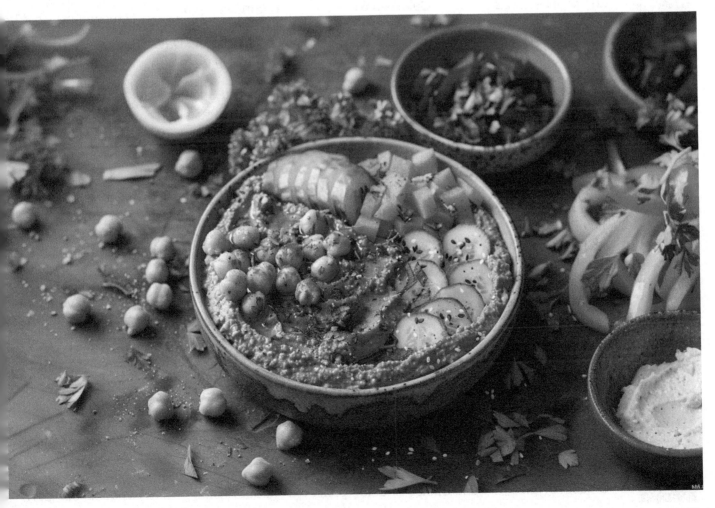

CHAPTER 2: 30-DAY MEAL PLAN

Day	Breakfast (600 kcal)	Lunch (600 kcal)	Snack (400 kcal)	Dinner (400 kcal)
Day 1	Greek Yogurt and Feta Omelette - p.20	Creamy Carrot and Ginger Soup - p.35	Avocado and Black Bean Stuffed Mini Peppers - p.50	Lemon Garlic Shrimp and Quinoa - p.66
Day 2	Mango and Turmeric Lassi - p.31	Quinoa and Black Bean Stuffed Peppers - p.37	Classic Hummus with Paprika - p.52	Mediterranean Eggplant Bake - p.69
Day 3	Curried Cauliflower and Egg Skillet - p.23	One-Pot Mediterranean Pasta with Olives - p.41	Coconut and Matcha Energy Bars - p.57	Lemon Garlic Chicken and Barley Salad - p.6
Day 4	Blueberry and Turmeric Oatmeal - p.27	Spicy Chickpea and Brown Rice Bowl - p.39	Baked Falafel Balls - p.55	Herb-Crusted Salmon with Asparagus - p.66
Day 5	Spinach and Ricotta Stuffed Crêpes - p.32	Tomato Basil and Quinoa Soup - p.35	Beet and Walnut Hummus with Crudités - p.51	BBQ Turkey Meatloaf with Cauliflower Rice p.74
Day 6	Zucchini and Bell Pepper Egg Muffins - p.22	Lentil and Bulgur Wheat Salad - p.61	Cucumber and Dill Greek Yogurt Dip - p.53	Baked Polenta with Marinara and Mushrooms - p.70
Day 7	Green Detox Smoothie with Kale and Pineapple - p.30	Mushroom and Wild Rice Pilaf - p.37	Almond Butter and Date Bars - p.59	Turmeric Roasted Cod with Veggies - p.67
Day 8	Asparagus and Goat Cheese Egg Bake - p.22	Pumpkin and Chickpea Soup with Turmeric - p.36	Quinoa and Spinach Stuffed Tomatoes - p.51	Ground Turkey and Veggie Stuffed Zucchini - p.73
Day 9	Avocado and Spinach Egg Scramble - p.20	One-Pot Green Bean and Potato Stew - p.43	Zucchini and Quinoa Bites - p.50	Freekeh and Roasted Root Vegetable Salad p.62
Day 10	Cottage Cheese and Berry Parfait - p.24	One-Pot Broccoli and Cheddar Quinoa - p.42	Chia Seed Pudding with Almonds and Blueberries - p.57	Ratatouille with Fresh Herbs - p.71
Day 11	Black Rice and Mango Porridge - p.29	Herb-Roasted Chicken with Quinoa Pilaf - p.45	Cauliflower Hash Browns with Poached Eggs - p.49	Lemon Basil Tilapia with Zucchini - p.68
Day 12	Veggie and Cheese Breakfast Quesadilla - p.32	Wild Rice and Cranberry Pilaf - p.38	Smoky Eggplant Baba Ganoush - p.53	Lentil and Vegetable Shepherd's Pie - p.70
Day 13	Mushroom and Swiss Chard Quiche - p.21	One-Pot Vegetable and Barley Casserole - p.41	Ginger and Turmeric Bliss Balls - p.58	Lemon Herb Chicken and Quinoa Salad - p.44
Day 14	Pumpkin Spice and Flaxseed Oatmeal - p.28	Couscous and Chickpea Pilaf - p.40	Artichoke and Spinach Yogurt Dip - p.54	Vegan Lasagna with Cashew Cheese - p.72
Day 15	Berry and Beetroot Smoothie - p.30	One-Pot Creamy Tomato and Spinach Pasta - p.43	Mini Avocado Toasts with Tomato - p.56	Balsamic Chicken and Vegetables - p.47

Day	Breakfast (600 kcal)	Lunch (600 kcal)	Snack (400 kcal)	Dinner (400 kcal)
Day 16	Turmeric Spiced Shakshuka - p.21	Spicy Turkey and Sweet Potato Skillet - p.44	Carrot and Cumin Fritters - p.50	Mediterranean Baked Fish with Olives and Tomatoes - p.67
Day 17	Banana and Almond Porridge - p.28	Green Lentil and Quinoa Stuffed Squash - p.40	Avocado and Cilantro Salsa - p.52	BBQ Chicken and Sweet Potato Wedges - p.72
Day 18	Spinach and Kiwi Green Juice - p.31	Quinoa and Black Bean Stuffed Peppers - p.37	Cashew and Herb Pesto - p.54	Baked Haddock with Tomato Relish - p.68
Day 19	Apple and Date Overnight Oats - p.29	Moroccan Spiced Turkey Meatballs - p.46	Roasted Red Pepper and Chickpea Crostini - p.50	Herb Marinated Pork Tenderloin with Asparagus - p.73
Day 20	Egg and Turkey Sausage Breakfast Muffins - p.33	Minestrone with Cannellini Beans and Kale - p.36	Sweet Potato and Kale Quesadillas - p.50	Anti-Inflammatory Paella - p.74
Day 21	Greek Yogurt Pancakes with Fresh Berries - p.32	Tomato Basil and Quinoa Soup - p.35	Spiced Sweet Potato and Cashew Bites - p.58	Spinach and Ricotta Stuffed Shells - p.71
Day 22	Sweet Potato and Kale Quesadillas - p.50	One-Pot Eggplant and Chickpea Tagine - p.42	Carrot and Cumin Fritters - p.50	Balsamic Chicken and Roasted Vegetables - p.47
Day 23	Lemon Poppy Seed Porridge - p.27	One-Pot Mediterranean Pasta with Olives - p.41	Classic Hummus with Paprika - p.52	Lentil and Vegetable Shepherd's Pie - p.70
Day 24	Broccoli and Cheddar Breakfast Casserole - p.23	Spicy Chickpea and Brown Rice Bowl - p.39	Quinoa and Spinach Stuffed Tomatoes - p.51	Herb-Crusted Salmon with Asparagus - p.66
Day 25	Mixed Berry and Almond Smoothie - p.30	Moroccan Spiced Turkey Meatballs - p.46	Mini Avocado Toasts with Tomato - p.56	Vegan Lasagna with Cashew Cheese - p.72
Day 26	Cranberry and Pecan Porridge - p.29	Green Lentil and Quinoa Stuffed Squash - p.40	Beet and Walnut Hummus with Crudités - p.51	Lemon Basil Tilapia with Zucchini - p.68
Day 27	Almond Flour Waffles with Cottage Cheese - p.26	Lentil and Bulgur Wheat Salad - p.61	Cucumber and Dill Greek Yogurt Dip - p.53	Baked Polenta with Marinara and Mushrooms - p.70
Day 28	Spinach and Mushroom Keto Quiche - p.23	Mushroom and Wild Rice Pilaf - p.37	Ginger and Turmeric Bliss Balls - p.58	BBQ Turkey Meatloaf with Cauliflower Rice - p.74
Day 29	Zucchini and Bell Pepper Egg Muffins - p.22	One-Pot Creamy Tomato and Spinach Pasta - p.43	Almond Butter and Date Bars - p.59	Ratatouille with Fresh Herbs - p.71
Day 30	Spinach and Kiwi Green Juice - p.31	Herb-Roasted Chicken with Quinoa Pilaf - p.45	Roasted Chickpeas with Paprika - p.52	Mediterranean Baked Fish with Olives and Tomatoes - p.67

Note: We wish to remind you that the 30-Day Meal Plan provided in this book serves as a guide and a source of inspiration. The caloric content of the dishes is approximate and may vary depending on portion sizes and specific ingredients. Our meal plan is designed to offer a diverse and balanced menu, rich in proteins, healthy fats, and carbohydrates, allowing you to maintain a healthy eating pattern without sacrificing the joy of enjoying delicious meals every day.

If you find that the calories in the recipes do not completely align with your personal needs or goals, feel free to adjust the portion sizes accordingly. Increase or decrease them to ensure the meal plan suits your individual preferences and dietary objectives. Be creative and enjoy each dish according to your needs!

Caloric Distribution:

- Breakfast (30% of total daily calories)
- Lunch (30% of total daily calories)
- Snack (20% of total daily calories)
- Dinner (20% of total daily calories)

By following these guidelines, you can enjoy a well-balanced diet that supports your health and wellness goals while savoring every bite.

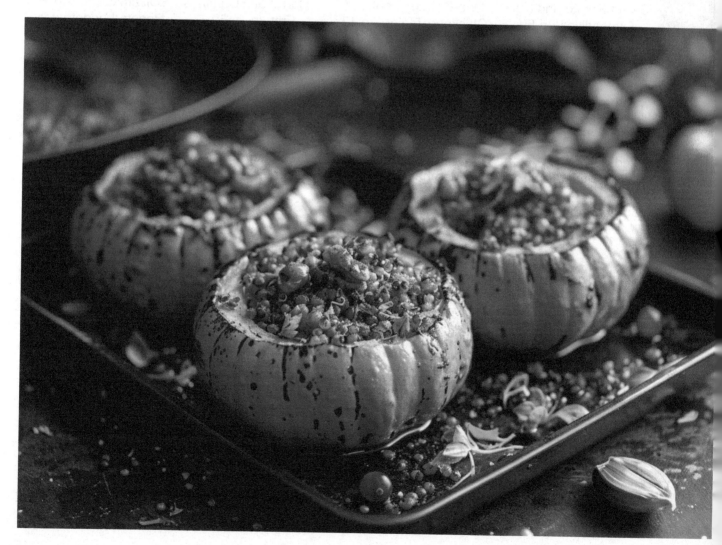

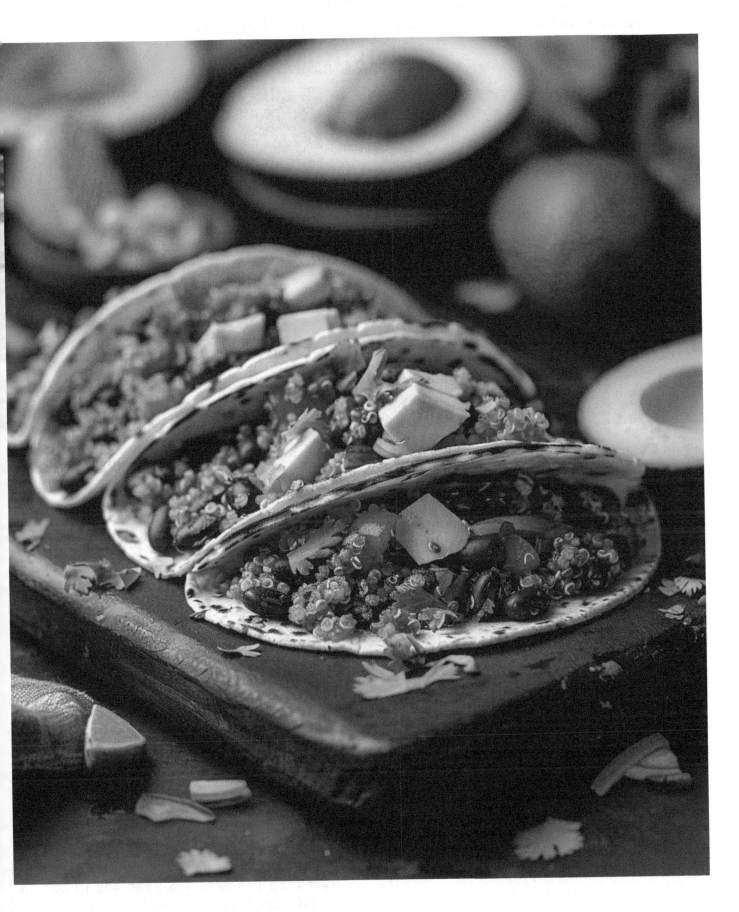

CHAPTER 3: BREAKFAST: Delicious Egg Dishes

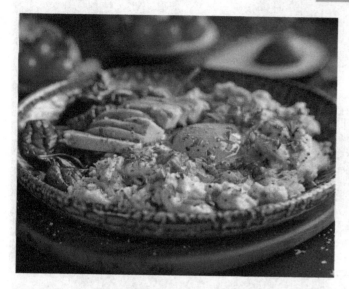

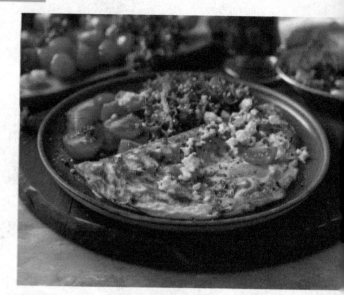

Avocado and Spinach Egg Scramble

Prep: 5 minutes | Cook: 10 minutes | Serves: 2

Ingredients:

- 4 large eggs (200g)
- 1/2 cup diced avocado (75g)
- 1 cup fresh spinach, chopped (30g)
- 1 tbsp olive oil (15 ml)
- 1/4 tsp salt, black pepper (1.5g, 0.6g)

Instructions:

1. Heat olive oil in a non-stick skillet over medium heat.
2. Add spinach and cook until wilted.
In a bowl, whisk eggs, salt, and pepper.
3. Pour the eggs into the skillet and gently scramble until almost set.
4. Add diced avocado and continue to cook until eggs are fully set. Garnish with egg yolk if desired.
5. Serve immediately.

Nutritional Facts (Per Serving): Calories: 600 | Carbs: 6g | Protein: 14g | Fat: 52g | Fiber: 4g | Sodium: 380 mg | Sugars: 1g

Greek Yogurt and Feta Omelette

Prep: 5 minutes | Cook: 10 minutes | Serves: 2

Ingredients:

- 4 large eggs (200g)
- 1/2 cup Greek yogurt (120g)
- 1/2 cup crumbled feta cheese (75g)
- 1 tbsp olive oil (15 ml)
- 1/4 cup chopped fresh parsley (15g)
- 1/4 tsp salt, black pepper (1.5g, 0.6g)

Instructions:

1. In a bowl, whisk eggs, Greek yogurt, salt, and pepper until smooth.
2. Heat olive oil in a non-stick skillet over medium heat.
3. Pour the egg mixture into the skillet, cook until eggs start to set.
4. Sprinkle feta cheese and parsley over half of the omelette.
5. Fold the omelette in half and cook until fully set.
6. Serve immediately.

Nutritional Facts (Per Serving): Calories: 600 | Carbs: 8g | Protein: 33g | Fat: 45g | Fiber: 1g | Sodium: 900 mg | Sugars: 4g

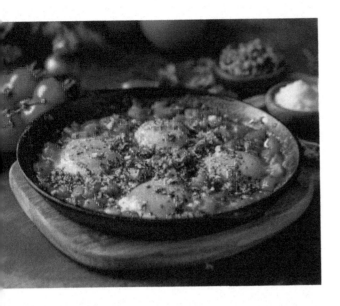

Turmeric Spiced Shakshuka

Prep: 10 minutes | Cook: 20 minutes | Serves: 2

Ingredients:

- 4 large eggs (200g)
- 1 can diced tomatoes (400g)
- 1 red bell pepper, onion, chopped (150g each)
- 2 cloves garlic, minced (8g)
- 1 tbsp olive oil (15 ml)
- 1 tsp ground turmeric, cumin (2.5g)
- 1/2 tsp paprika (1g)
- 1/4 tsp salt, black pepper (1.5g, 0.6g)
- Fresh cilantro for garnish (10g)

Instructions:

1. Heat olive oil in a large skillet over medium heat.
2. Add onion and bell pepper, cook until softened.
3. Add garlic, turmeric, cumin, paprika, salt, and pepper, cook for 1 minute.
4. Add diced tomatoes and simmer for 10 minutes.
5. Create wells in the tomato mixture and crack an egg into each well.
6. Cover and cook until eggs are set to your liking.
7. Garnish with fresh cilantro and serve.

Nutritional Facts (Per Serving): Calories: 600 | Carbs: 24g | Protein: 18g | Fat: 42g | Fiber: 7g | Sodium: 780 mg | Sugars: 12g

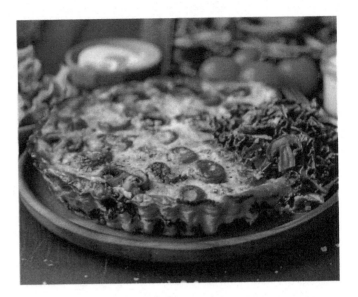

Mushroom and Swiss Chard Quiche

Prep: 5 minutes | Cook: 15 minutes | Serves: 2

Ingredients:

- 6 large eggs (300g)
- 1 cup heavy cream (250 ml)
- 1 cup chopped Swiss chard (50g)
- 1 cup sliced mushrooms (90g)
- 1 cup shredded Swiss cheese (100g)
- 1/2 tsp salt (3g)
- 1 tbsp butter (for greasing)

Instructions:

1. Preheat the oven to 375 °F (190 °C) and grease a pie dish with butter.
2. Sauté mushrooms and Swiss chard in a pan until cooked, then set aside to cool.
3. Whisk together eggs, cream, salt, and pepper.
4. Stir in the cooled mushrooms, Swiss chard, and cheese.
5. Pour into the prepared pie dish and bake until set and golden on top, about 35 minutes.
6. Slice and serve.

Nutritional Facts (Per Serving): Calories: 600 | Carbs: 8g | Protein: 27g | Fat: 50g | Fiber: 2g | Sodium: 700 mg | Sugars: 3g

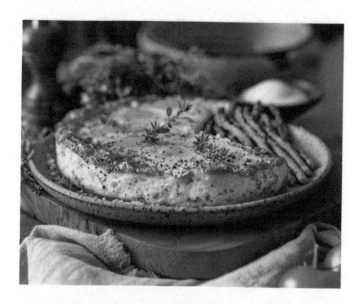

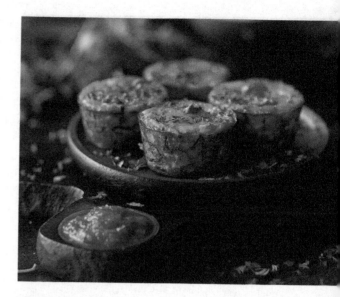

Asparagus and Goat Cheese Egg Bake

Prep: 10 minutes | Cook: 30 minutes | Serves: 2

Ingredients:

- 6 large eggs (300g)
- 1/2 cup heavy cream (120 ml)
- 1 cup chopped asparagus (150g)
- 1/2 cup crumbled goat cheese (75g)
- 1 tbsp olive oil (15 ml)
- 1/4 tsp salt, black pepper (1.5g, 0.6g)

Instructions:

1. Preheat the oven to 375 °F (190 °C) and grease a baking dish with olive oil.
2. In a bowl, whisk together eggs, heavy cream, salt, and pepper.
3. Add chopped asparagus and crumbled goat cheese to the egg mixture.
4. Pour the mixture into the prepared baking dish.
5. Bake for 30 minutes, or until set and golden on top. Slice and serve.

Nutritional Facts (Per Serving): Calories: 600 | Carbs: 7g | Protein: 24g | Fat: 50g | Fiber: 2g | Sodium: 450 mg | Sugars: 3g

Zucchini and Bell Pepper Egg Muffins

Prep: 10 minutes | Cook: 20 minutes | Serves: 2

Ingredients:

- 4 large eggs (200g)
- 1 cup grated zucchini (130g)
- 1/2 cup chopped red bell pepper (75g)
- 1/2 cup shredded cheddar cheese (60g)
- 1 tbsp olive oil (15 ml)
- 1/4 tsp salt, black pepper (1.5g, 0.6g)

Instructions:

1. Preheat the oven to 350 °F (180 °C) and grease a muffin tin with olive oil.
2. In a bowl, whisk together eggs, salt, and pepper.
3. Stir in grated zucchini, chopped bell pepper, and shredded cheese.
4. Divide the mixture evenly among the muffin cups.
5. Bake for 20 minutes, or until fully set.
6. Remove from the oven, let cool slightly, and serve.

Nutritional Facts (Per Serving): Calories: 600 | Carbs: 8g | Protein: 28g | Fat: 47g | Fiber: 2g | Sodium: 480 mg | Sugars: 4g

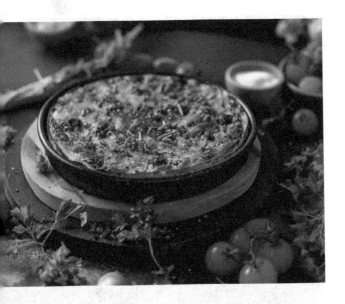

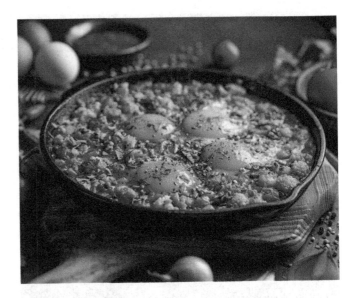

Broccoli and Cheddar Breakfast Casserole

Prep: 10 minutes | Cook: 35 minutes | Serves: 2

Ingredients:

- 6 large eggs (300g)
- 1 cup heavy cream (250 ml)
- 1 cup chopped broccoli (150g)
- 1 cup shredded cheddar cheese (100g)
- 1 tbsp olive oil (15 ml)
- 1/2 tsp salt, black pepper (1.5g, 0.6g)

Instructions:

1. Preheat the oven to 375 °F (190 °C) and grease a baking dish with olive oil.
2. In a bowl, whisk together eggs, heavy cream, salt, and pepper.
3. Add chopped broccoli and shredded cheddar cheese to the egg mixture.
4. Pour the mixture into the prepared baking dish.
5. Bake for 35 minutes, or until set and golden on top.
6. Slice and serve.

Nutritional Facts (Per Serving): Calories: 600 | Carbs: 9g | Protein: 28g | Fat: 49g | Fiber: 3g | Sodium: 600 mg | Sugars: 3g

Curried Cauliflower and Egg Skillet

Prep: 10 minutes | Cook: 20 minutes | Serves: 2

Ingredients:

- 4 large eggs (200g)
- 2 cups cauliflower florets (200g)
- 1 medium onion, chopped (150g)
- 1 tbsp olive oil (15 ml)
- 1 tsp curry powder (2g)
- 1/2 tsp ground cumin (1g)
- 1/4 tsp salt, black pepper (1.5g, 0.6g)
- Fresh cilantro for garnish (10g)

Instructions:

1. Heat olive oil in a skillet over medium heat.
2. Add chopped onion and sauté until translucent.
3. Add cauliflower florets, curry powder, cumin, salt, and pepper. Cook until cauliflower is tender.
4. Create wells in the cauliflower mixture and crack an egg into each well.
5. Cover and cook until eggs are set to your liking.
6. Garnish with fresh cilantro and serve/

Nutritional Facts (Per Serving): Calories: 600 | Carbs: 14g | Protein: 20g | Fat: 50g | Fiber: 5g | Sodium: 500 mg | Sugars: 6g

CHAPTER 4: BREAKFASTS: Protein-Packed

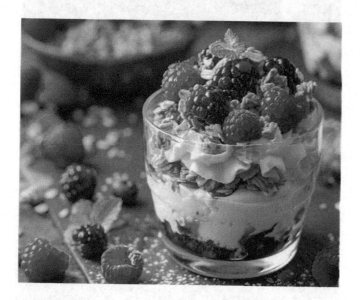

Cottage Cheese and Berry Parfait

Prep: 5 minutes | Cook: 0 minutes | Serves: 2

Ingredients:

- 1 cup cottage cheese (240g)
- 1 cup mixed berries (150g)
- 2 tbsp low-carb sweeteners (30g)
- 1/4 cup granola (30g

Instructions:

1. In two serving glasses, layer cottage cheese, mixed berries, and low-carb sweeteners.
2. Top with granola.
3. Serve immediately.

Nutritional Facts (Per Serving): Calories: 600 | Carbs: 30g | Protein: 28g | Fat: 30g | Fiber: 5g | Sodium: 400 mg | Sugars: 15g

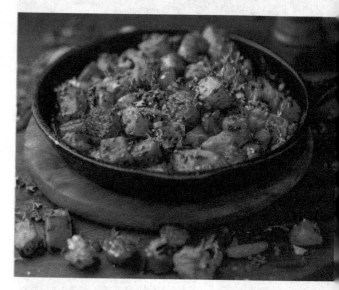

Turkey Sausage and Sweet Potato Hash

Prep: 10 minutes | Cook: 20 minutes | Serves: 2

Ingredients:

- 1/2 lb ground turkey sausage (225g)
- 1 large sweet potato, diced (200g)
- 1 red bell pepper, chopped (150g)
- 1 small onion, chopped (100g)
- 2 tbsp olive oil (30 ml)
- 1/2 tsp salt, black pepper (1.5g, 0.6g)

Instructions:

1. Heat olive oil in a large skillet over medium heat.
2. Add diced sweet potato and cook until tender.
3. Add onion and bell pepper, cook until softened.
4. Add turkey sausage, cook until browned.
5. Season with salt and pepper.
6. Serve immediately

Nutritional Facts (Per Serving): Calories: 600 | Carbs: 30g | Protein: 30g | Fat: 35g | Fiber: 5g | Sodium: 800 mg | Sugars: 8g

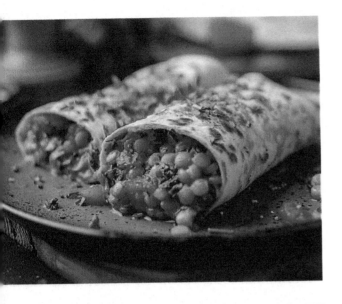

Lentil and Veggie Breakfast Wrap

Prep: 10 minutes | Cook: 10 minutes | Serves: 2

Ingredients:

- 1/2 cup cooked lentils (100g)
- 1/2 cup chopped spinach (30g)
- 1/2 cup diced tomatoes (75g)
- 1/4 cup shredded carrot (30g)
- 2 whole grain tortillas (60g each)
- 2 tbsp hummus (30g)
- 1 tbsp olive oil (15 ml)
- 1/4 tsp salt, black pepper (1.5g, 0.6g)

Instructions:

1. In a skillet, heat olive oil over medium heat.
2. Add spinach, tomatoes, and carrots, cook until tender.
3. Stir in cooked lentils, salt, and pepper, cook until heated through.
4. Spread hummus on each tortilla, add the lentil mixture, and wrap.
5. Serve immediately.

Nutritional Facts (Per Serving): Calories: 600 | Carbs: 80g | Protein: 20g | Fat: 20g | Fiber: 12g | Sodium: 600 mg | Sugars: 6g

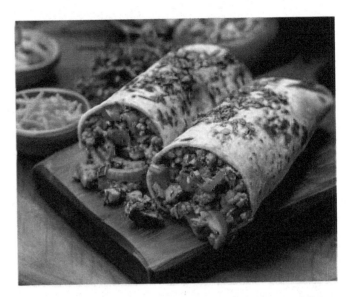

Turkey and Veggie Breakfast Burrito

Prep: 10 minutes | Cook: 10 minutes | Serves: 2

Ingredients:

- 1/2 lb ground turkey (225g)
- 1/2 cup diced bell pepper, zucchini (75g each)
- 1 small onion, chopped (100g)
- 2 whole grain tortillas (60g)
- 1/2 cup shredded cheddar cheese (60g)
- 2 tbsp olive oil (30 ml)
- 1/2 tsp salt (3g)
- 1/4 tsp black pepper (0.6g)

Instructions:

1. Heat olive oil in a skillet over medium heat.
2. Add onion, bell pepper, and zucchini, cook until tender.
3. Add ground turkey, cook until browned.
4. Season with salt and pepper.
5. Divide the mixture between the tortillas, top with cheddar cheese, and wrap.
6. Serve immediately.

Nutritional Facts (Per Serving): Calories: 600 | Carbs: 35g | Protein: 35g | Fat: 30g | Fiber: 5g | Sodium: 700 mg | Sugars:5g

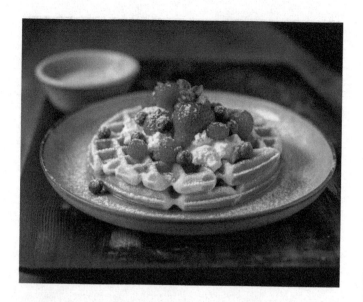

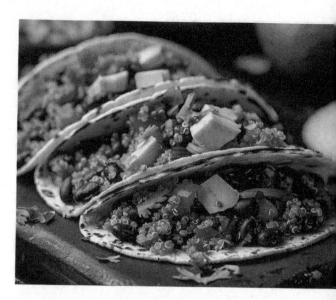

Almond Flour Waffles with Cottage Cheese

Prep: 10 minutes | Cook: 15 minutes | Serves: 2

Ingredients:

- 1 cup almond flour (96g)
- 1/2 tsp baking powder (2g)
- 1/4 tsp salt (1.5g)
- 2 large eggs (100g)
- 1/2 cup cottage cheese (120g)
- 2 tbsp almond milk (30 ml)
- 1 tbsp melted butter (15g)
- 1 tbsp low-carb sweeteners (15g)

Instructions:

1. Preheat the waffle iron.
2. In a bowl, mix almond flour, baking powder, and salt.
3. In another bowl, whisk eggs, cottage cheese, almond milk, melted butter, and low-carb sweeteners.
4. Combine wet and dry ingredients, mix until smooth.
5. Pour batter into the preheated waffle iron, cook until golden brown.
6. Serve with your favorite toppings.

Nutritional Facts (Per Serving): Calories: 600 | Carbs: 8g | Protein: 28g | Fat: 50g | Fiber: 4g | Sodium: 500 mg | Sugars: 3g

Black Bean and Quinoa Breakfast Tacos

Prep: 10 minutes | Cook: 15 minutes | Serves: 2

Ingredients:

- 1/2 cup cooked quinoa (90g)
- 1/2 cup black beans, drained and rinsed (85g)
- 1/2 cup diced tomatoes (75g)
- 1/4 cup chopped cilantro (15g)
- 1/4 cup diced red onion (35g)
- 1/2 avocado, sliced (75g)
- 2 whole grain tortillas (60g)
- 1 tbsp olive oil (15 ml)
- 1/2 tsp ground cumin (1g)
- 1/4 tsp salt, black pepper (1.5g, 0.6g)

Instructions:

1. Heat olive oil in a skillet over medium heat.
2. Add diced red onion and cook until translucent.
3. Add quinoa, black beans, tomatoes, ground cumin, salt, and pepper. Cook until heated through.
4. Warm tortillas in a separate pan or microwave.
5. Divide the quinoa mixture between the tortillas, top with avocado slices and chopped cilantro.
6. Serve immediately.

Nutritional Facts (Per Serving): Calories: 600 | Carbs: 70g | Protein: 18g | Fat: 28g | Fiber: 16g | Sodium: 400 mg | Sugars: 5g

CHAPTER 5: BREAKFASTS: Anti-Inflammatory Oatmeals and Porridges

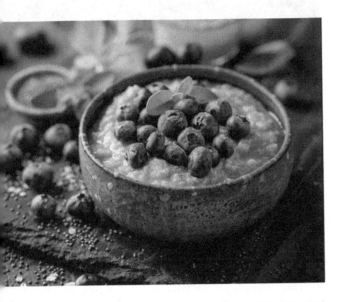

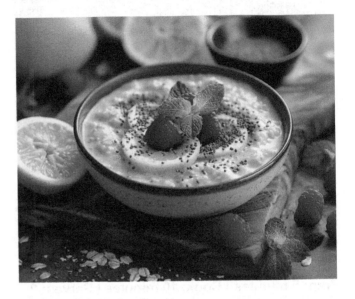

Blueberry and Turmeric Oatmeal

Prep: 5 minutes | Cook: 10 minutes | Serves: 2

Ingredients:

- 1 cup rolled oats (90g)
- 2 cups almond milk (480 ml)
- 1 cup fresh blueberries (150g)
- 1 tbsp low-carb sweeteners (15g)
- 1 tsp ground turmeric (2g)
- 1/2 tsp ground cinnamon (1.2g)
- 1/4 tsp salt (1.5g)
- 1 tbsp chia seeds (12g)

Instructions:

1. In a saucepan, bring almond milk to a simmer.
2. Add rolled oats, ground turmeric, ground cinnamon, and salt. Cook for 5-7 minutes, stirring occasionally.
3. Stir in low-carb sweeteners and chia seeds.
4. Remove from heat and fold in fresh blueberries.
5. Serve immediately.

Nutritional Facts (Per Serving): Calories: 600 | Carbs: 75g | Protein: 15g | Fat: 25g | Fiber: 10g | Sodium: 300 mg | Sugars: 10g

Lemon Poppy Seed Porridge

Prep: 5 minutes | Cook: 10 minutes | Serves: 2

Ingredients:

- 1 cup rolled oats (90g)
- 2 cups almond milk (480 ml)
- 1 tbsp poppy seeds (10g)
- 1 tbsp low-carb sweeteners (15g)
- 1 tsp lemon zest (2g)
- 1 tbsp lemon juice (15 ml)
- 1/4 tsp salt (1.5g)

Instructions:

1. In a saucepan, bring almond milk to a simmer.
2. Add rolled oats, poppy seeds, low-carb sweeteners, lemon zest, lemon juice, and salt.
3. Cook for 5-7 minutes, stirring occasionally, until thickened.
4. Serve warm.

Nutritional Facts (Per Serving): Calories: 600 | Carbs: 80g | Protein: 15g | Fat: 20g | Fiber: 10g | Sodium: 300 mg | Sugars: 10g

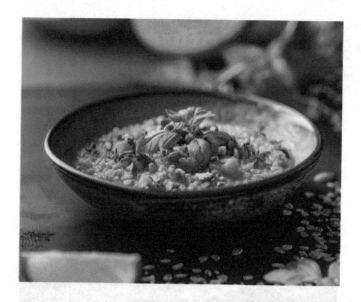

Pumpkin Spice and Flaxseed Oatmeal

Prep: 5 minutes | Cook: 10 minutes | Serves: 2

Ingredients:

- 1 cup rolled oats (90g)
- 2 cups almond milk (480 ml)
- 1/2 cup pumpkin purée (120g)
- 1 tbsp flaxseed meal (7g)
- 1 tbsp low-carb sweeteners (15g)
- 1 tsp pumpkin spice (2g)
- 1/4 tsp salt (1.5g)

Instructions:

1. In a saucepan, bring almond milk to a simmer.
2. Add rolled oats, pumpkin purée, flaxseed meal, low-carb sweeteners, pumpkin spice, and salt.
3. Cook for 5-7 minutes, stirring occasionally, until thickened.
4. Serve warm.

Nutritional Facts (Per Serving): Calories: 600 | Carbs: 75g | Protein: 15g | Fat: 25g | Fiber: 10g | Sodium: 300 mg | Sugars: 10g

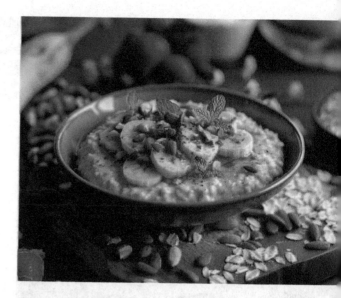

Banana and Almond Porridge

Prep: 5 minutes | Cook: 10 minutes | Serves: 2

Ingredients:

- 1 cup rolled oats (90g)
- 2 cups almond milk (480 ml)
- 1 ripe banana, mashed (120g)
- 2 tbsp almond butter (32g)
- 1 tbsp low-carb sweeteners (15g)
- 1/4 tsp salt (1.5g)
- 1/2 tsp ground cinnamon (1g)

Instructions:

1. In a saucepan, bring almond milk to a simmer.
2. Add rolled oats, mashed banana, almond butter, low-carb sweeteners, salt, and cinnamon.
3. Cook for 5-7 minutes, stirring occasionally, until thickened.
4. Serve warm.

Nutritional Facts (Per Serving): Calories: 600 | Carbs: 80g | Protein: 15g | Fat: 25g | Fiber: 10g | Sodium: 300 mg | Sugars: 20g

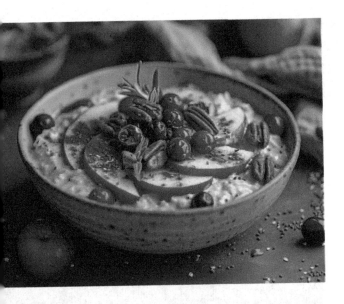

Cranberry and Pecan Porridge with Apple and Date Overnight Oats

Prep: 10 minutes | Cook: overnight | Serves: 2

Ingredients:

- 1 cup rolled oats (90g)
- 1 cup unsweetened almond milk (240 ml)
- 1/2 cup diced apple (75g)
- 1/4 cup dried cranberries, chopped pecans (30g each)
- 2 dates, chopped (20g)
- 1 tbsp chia seeds (12g)
- 1 tbsp low-carb sweeteners (15g)
- 1/4 tsp ground cinnamon (1g)

Instructions:

1. In a bowl, combine rolled oats, almond milk, diced apple, dried cranberries, chopped pecans, chopped dates, chia seeds, low-carb sweeteners, and ground cinnamon.
2. Mix well and divide between two jars or containers.
3. Cover and refrigerate overnight.
4. Serve chilled in the morning, at lunch or before bed.

Nutritional Facts (Per Serving): Calories: 600 | Carbs: 85g | Protein: 10g | Fat: 25g | Fiber: 12g | Sodium: 150 mg | Sugars: 30g

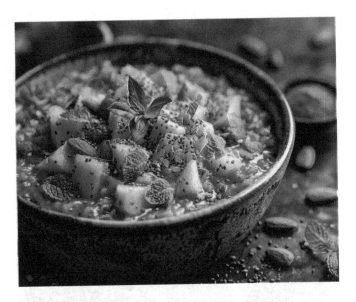

Black Rice and Mango Porridge

Prep: 10 minutes | Cook: 45 minutes | Serves: 2

Ingredients:

- 1/2 cup black rice (100g)
- 1 1/2 cups water (375ml)
- 1 cup unsweetened almond milk (250ml)
- 1 ripe mango, diced (200g)
- 1 tbsp low carb sweetener
- 1 tsp vanilla extract
- 1/4 tsp ground cinnamon
- 1/4 cup chopped almonds (30g)
- 1 tbsp chia seeds (15g)
- 1/4 tsp salt

Instructions:

1. Rinse the black rice under cold water until the water runs clear.
2. In a medium saucepan, combine the black rice, water, and salt. Bring to a boil over medium-high heat, then reduce the heat to low, cover, and simmer for 30 minutes.
3. Stir in the almond milk, low carb sweetener, vanilla extract, and ground cinnamon. Continue to simmer for another 10-15 minutes, or until the rice is tender and the mixture is creamy.
4. Remove from heat and let sit for 5 minutes.
5. Serve the porridge topped with diced mango, chopped almonds, and chia seeds.

Nutritional Facts (Per Serving): Calories: 600 | Carbs: 90g | Protein: 12g | Fat: 22g | Fiber: 10g | Sodium: 300mg | Sugars: 20g

CHAPTER 6: BREAKFASTS: Energizing Smoothies and Juices

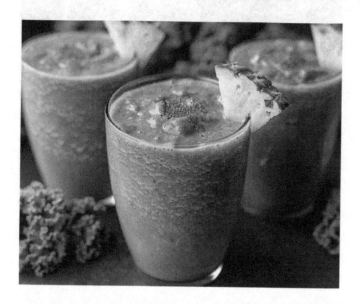

Green Detox Smoothie with Kale and Pineapple

Prep: 5 minutes | Cook: 0 minutes | Serves: 2

Ingredients:

- 1 cup kale, chopped (30g)
- 1 cup fresh pineapple, diced (165g)
- 1 banana (120g)
- 1 cup unsweetened almond milk (240 ml)
- 1 tbsp chia seeds (12g)
- 1 tbsp low-carb sweeteners (15g)

Instructions:

1. Combine kale, pineapple, banana, almond milk, chia seeds, and low-carb sweeteners in a blender.
2. Blend until smooth.
3. Serve immediately.

Nutritional Facts (Per Serving): Calories: 600 | Carbs: 85g | Protein: 10g | Fat: 25g | Fiber: 12g | Sodium: 150 mg | Sugars: 40g

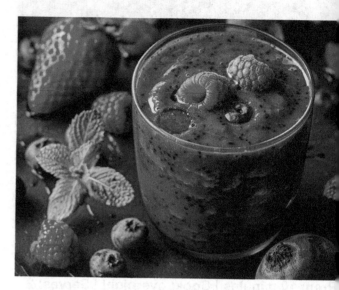

Berry and Beetroot Smoothie

Prep: 5 minutes | Cook: 0 minutes | Serves: 2

Ingredients:

- 1 cup mixed berries (150g)
- 1 small beetroot, peeled and diced (100g)
- 1 banana (120g)
- 1 cup unsweetened almond milk (240 ml)
- 1 tbsp low-carb sweeteners (15g)

Instructions:

1. Combine mixed berries, beetroot, banana, almond milk, and low-carb sweeteners in a blender.
2. Blend until smooth.
3. Serve immediately.

Nutritional Facts (Per Serving): Calories: 600 | Carbs: 90g | Protein: 8g | Fat: 15g | Fiber: 12g | Sodium: 100 mg | Sugars: 50g

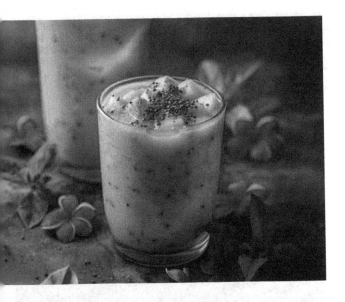

Mango and Turmeric Lassi

Prep: 5 minutes | Cook: 0 minutes | Serves: 2

Ingredients:

- 1 cup fresh mango, diced (165g)
- 1 cup Greek yogurt (240g)
- 1 cup unsweetened almond milk (240 ml)
- 1 tsp ground turmeric (2g)
- 1 tbsp low-carb sweeteners (15g)
- 1/4 tsp ground cardamom (0.5g)

Instructions:

1. Combine mango, Greek yogurt, almond milk, turmeric, low-carb sweeteners, and ground cardamom in a blender.
2. Blend until smooth.
3. Serve immediately.

Nutritional Facts (Per Serving): Calories: 600 | Carbs: 80g | Protein: 20g | Fat: 20g | Fiber: 5g | Sodium: 150 mg | Sugars: 60g

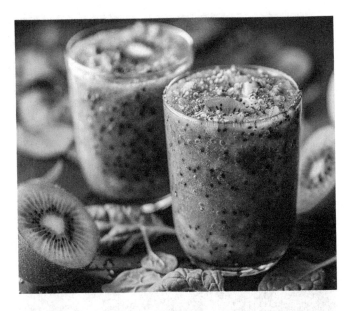

Spinach and Kiwi Green Juice

Prep: 5 minutes | Cook: 0 minutes | Serves: 2

Ingredients:

- 1 cup fresh spinach (30g)
- 2 kiwis, peeled (140g)
- 1 apple, cored and chopped (180g)
- 1 cup unsweetened coconut water (240 ml)
- 1 tbsp low-carb sweeteners (15g)
- 1 tbsp fresh lime juice (15 ml)

Instructions:

1. Combine spinach, kiwis, apple, coconut water, low-carb sweeteners, and lime juice in a blender.
2. Blend until smooth.
3. Serve immediately.

Nutritional Facts (Per Serving): Calories: 600 | Carbs: 95g | Protein: 5g | Fat: 15g | Fiber: 10g | Sodium: 100 mg | Sugars: 70g

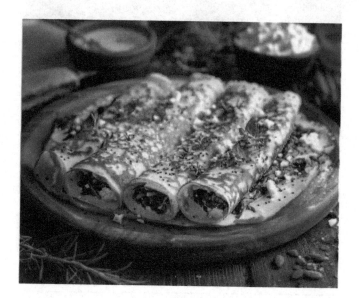

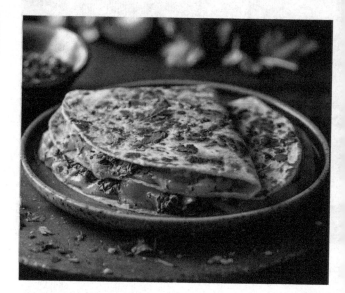

Spinach and Ricotta Stuffed Crêpes

Prep: 10 minutes | Cook: 20 minutes | Serves: 2

Ingredients:

- 1 cup whole wheat flour (120g)
- 1 1/4 cups almond milk (300 ml)
- 2 large eggs (100g)
- 1 tbsp olive oil (15 ml)
- 1/2 cup ricotta cheese (125g)
- 1 cup fresh spinach, chopped (30g)
- 1/4 tsp salt (1.5g)
- 1/4 tsp black pepper (0.6g)

Instructions:

1. In a bowl, whisk flour, almond milk, eggs, and olive oil until smooth.
2. Heat a non-stick skillet over medium heat and pour in a small amount of batter, swirling to coat the bottom. Cook for 2-3 minutes on each side until golden, then set aside.
3. In another bowl, mix ricotta, spinach, salt, and pepper. Spoon the mixture onto each crêpe, roll up, and serve.

Nutritional Facts (Per Serving): Calories: 600 | Carbs: 50g | Protein: 20g | Fat: 34g | Fiber: 8g | Sodium: 600 mg | Sugars: 5g

Veggie and Cheese Breakfast Quesadilla

Prep: 10 minutes | Cook: 10 minutes | Serves: 2

Ingredients:

- 2 whole grain tortillas (60g each)
- 1/2 cup shredded cheddar cheese (60g)
- 1/2 cup chopped bell peppers, zucchini (75g each)
- 1/2 cup chopped spinach (30g)
- 1 tbsp olive oil (15 ml)
- 1/4 tsp salt (1.5g)
- 1/4 tsp black pepper (0.6g)

Instructions:

1. Heat olive oil in a skillet over medium heat.
2. Add bell peppers and spinach, cook until tender.
3. Place one tortilla in the skillet, sprinkle half of the cheese, add the veggies, then the remaining cheese, and top with the second tortilla.
4. Cook until golden brown and the cheese is melted, flipping once. Slice and serve.

Nutritional Facts (Per Serving): Calories: 600 | Carbs: 45g | Protein: 20g | Fat: 35g | Fiber: 8g | Sodium: 500 mg | Sugars: 4g

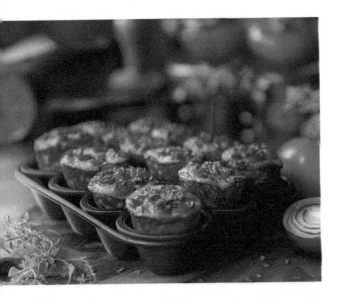

Egg and Turkey Sausage Breakfast Muffins

Prep: 10 minutes | Cook: 20 minutes | Serves: 2

Ingredients:

- 4 large eggs (200g)
- 1/2 cup cooked and crumbled turkey sausage (85g)
- 1/4 cup diced bell pepper, onion (35g each)
- 1/4 cup shredded cheddar cheese (30g)
- 1 tbsp olive oil (15 ml)
- 1/4 tsp salt, black pepper (1.5g, 0.6g)

Instructions:

1. Preheat the oven to 350 °F (180 °C) and grease a muffin tin with olive oil.
2. In a bowl, whisk together eggs, salt, and pepper.
3. Add turkey sausage, bell pepper, onion, and cheese, mix well.
4. Pour the mixture evenly into the muffin tin.
5. Bake for 20 minutes, or until fully set.
6. Serve warm.

Nutritional Facts (Per Serving): Calories: 600 | Carbs: 6g | Protein: 35g | Fat: 45g | Fiber: 1g | Sodium: 700 mg | Sugars: 2g

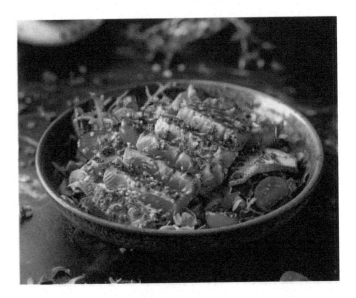

Seared Tuna and Avocado Breakfast Salad

Prep: 10 minutes | Cook: 5 minutes | Serves: 2

Ingredients:

- 2 tuna steaks (200g each)
- 1 avocado, sliced (150g)
- 4 cups mixed greens (120g)
- 1/2 cup cherry tomatoes, halved (75g)
- 1/4 cup red onion, thinly sliced (35g)
- 2 tbsp olive oil (30 ml)
- 1 tbsp lemon juice (15 ml)
- 1/4 tsp salt, black pepper (1.5g, 0.6g)

Instructions:

1. Heat 1 tbsp olive oil in a skillet over high heat.
2. Season tuna steaks with salt and pepper, sear for 1-2 minutes per side.
3. In a bowl, combine mixed greens, avocado, cherry tomatoes, and red onion.
4. Whisk together remaining olive oil and lemon juice, drizzle over salad.
5. Top with seared tuna slices and serve.

Nutritional Facts (Per Serving): Calories: 600 | Carbs: 12g | Protein: 40g | Fat: 45g | Fiber: 7g | Sodium: 450 mg | Sugars: 4g

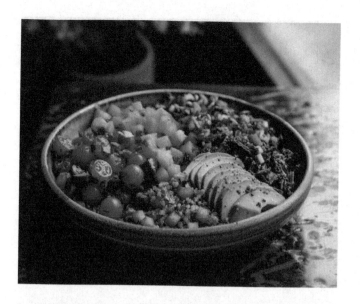

Quinoa and Vegetable Breakfast Bowl

Prep 10 minutes | Cook: 15 minutes | Serves: 2

Ingredients:

- 1 cup cooked quinoa (170g)
- 1/2 cup chopped bell pepper (75g)
- 1/2 cup chopped zucchini (75g)
- 1/2 cup cherry tomatoes, halved (75g)
- 1/4 cup chopped red onion (37g)
- 1/2 avocado, sliced (75g)
- 1 tbsp olive oil (15 ml)
- 1 tbsp lemon juice (15 ml)
- 1/4 tsp salt (1.5g)
- 1/4 tsp black pepper (0.6g)

Instructions:

1. Heat olive oil in a skillet over medium heat.
2. Add bell pepper, zucchini, and red onion, cook until tender.
3. In a bowl, combine cooked quinoa, sautéed vegetables, cherry tomatoes, lemon juice, salt, and pepper.
4. Top with avocado slices and serve.

Nutritional Facts (Per Serving): Calories: 600 | Carbs: 70g | Protein: 15g | Fat: 30g | Fiber: 12g | Sodium: 400 mg | Sugars: 6g

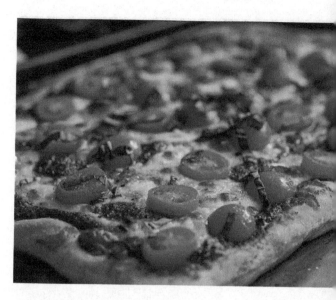

Pesto and Tomato Breakfast Pizza

Prep: 10 minutes | Cook: 15 minutes | Serves: 2

Ingredients:

- 1 whole wheat pizza crust (200g)
- 1/2 cup pesto sauce (120g)
- 1 cup cherry tomatoes, halved (150g)
- 1/2 cup shredded mozzarella cheese (60g)
- 2 tbsp grated Parmesan cheese (20g)
- 1 tbsp olive oil (15 ml)
- 1/4 tsp salt (1.5g)
- 1/4 tsp black pepper (0.6g)

Instructions:

1. Preheat the oven to 425 °F (220 °C).
2. Place pizza crust on a baking sheet.
3. Spread pesto sauce evenly over the crust.
4. Top with cherry tomatoes, mozzarella cheese, and grated Parmesan cheese.
5. Drizzle with olive oil, sprinkle with salt and black pepper.
6. Bake for 12-15 minutes, until cheese is melted and crust is golden brown.
7. Slice and serve.

Nutritional Facts (Per Serving): Calories: 600 | Carbs: 45g | Protein: 18g | Fat: 40g | Fiber: 5g | Sodium: 700 mg | Sugars: 3g

CHAPTER 8: LUNCHES: Hearty Soups and Stews

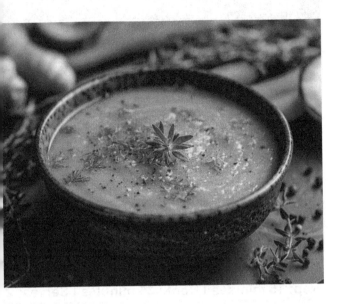

Creamy Carrot and Ginger Soup

Prep: 10 minutes | Cook: 25 minutes | Serves: 2

Ingredients:

- 2 tbsp olive oil (30 ml)
- 1 small onion, chopped (100g)
- 4 large carrots, sliced (500g)
- 1 tbsp fresh ginger, grated (15g)
- 3 cups vegetable broth (720 ml)
- 1/2 cup coconut milk (120 ml)
- 1/2 tsp salt (2.5g)
- 1/4 tsp black pepper (1g)

Instructions:

1. Heat olive oil in a pot over medium heat. Add onion and sauté until translucent.
2. Add carrots and ginger, cook for 5 minutes.
3. Pour in the vegetable broth and bring to a boil.
4. Reduce heat and simmer until carrots are tender, about 20 minutes.
5. Blend the soup until smooth. Stir in coconut milk, salt, and pepper. Serve hot.

Nutritional Facts (Per Serving): Calories: 600 | Carbs: 40g | Protein: 6g | Fat: 42g | Fiber: 10g | Sodium: 1200 mg | Sugars: 12g

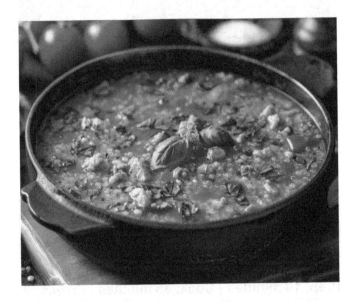

Tomato Basil and Quinoa Soup

Prep: 15 minutes | Cook: 30 minutes | Serves: 2

Ingredients:

- 2 tbsp olive oil (30 ml)
- 1 small onion, chopped (100g)
- 3 cloves garlic, minced (9g)
- 1 can diced tomatoes (400g)
- 3 cups vegetable broth (720 ml)
- 1/2 cup quinoa, rinsed (90g)
- 1/2 cup fresh basil, chopped (15g)
- 1/2 tsp salt (2.5g)
- 1/4 tsp black pepper (1g)

Instructions:

1. Heat olive oil in a pot over medium heat. Add onion and garlic, sauté until fragrant.
2. Add diced tomatoes and vegetable broth, bring to a boil.
3. Stir in quinoa, reduce heat, and simmer for 20 minutes.
4. Add fresh basil, salt, and pepper, simmer for another 5 minutes. Serve hot.

Nutritional Facts (Per Serving): Calories: 600 | Carbs: 60g | Protein: 12g | Fat: 30g | Fiber: 10g | Sodium: 1000 mg | Sugars: 12g

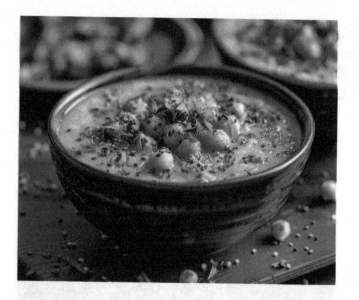

Pumpkin and Chickpea Soup with Turmeric

Prep: 10 minutes | Cook: 35 minutes | Serves: 2

Ingredients:

- 2 tbsp olive oil (30 ml)
- 1 small onion, chopped (100g)
- 3 cloves garlic, minced (9g)
- 2 cups pumpkin puree (450g)
- 1 can chickpeas, drained (240g)
- 3 cups vegetable broth (720 ml)
- 1 tsp turmeric (5g)
- 1/2 cup coconut milk (120 ml)
- 1/2 tsp salt (2.5g)
- 1/4 tsp black pepper (1g)

Instructions:

1. Heat olive oil in a large pot over medium heat. Sauté onion and garlic until translucent, about 5 minutes.

2. Add turmeric and stir for 1 minute. Add pumpkin purée, chickpeas, and vegetable broth. Bring to a boil, then reduce heat and simmer for 20 minutes.

3. Use an immersion blender to puree the soup until smooth.

4. Stir in coconut milk and season with salt and pepper. Heat through.

Nutritional Facts (Per Serving): Calories: 600 | Carbs: 55g | Protein: 12g | Fat: 35g | Fiber: 14g | Sodium: 1100 mg | Sugars: 10g

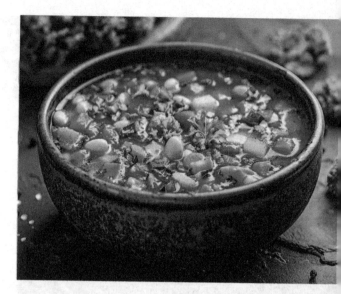

Minestrone with Cannellini Beans and Kale

Prep: 15 minutes | Cook: 35 minutes | Serves: 2

Ingredients:

- 2 tbsp olive oil (30 ml)
- 1 small onion, chopped (100g)
- 2 cloves garlic, minced (6g)
- 2 carrots, diced (250g)
- 1 zucchini, diced (200g)
- 1 can diced tomatoes (400g)
- 3 cups vegetable broth (720 ml)
- 1 can cannellini beans, drained (240g)
- 1 cup kale, chopped (70g)
- 1 tsp dried oregano, black pepper, (1g each)
- 1/2 tsp salt (2.5g

Instructions:

1. Heat olive oil in a pot over medium heat. Add onion and garlic, sauté until fragrant.

2. Add carrots and zucchini, cook for 5 minutes.

3. Stir in diced tomatoes, vegetable broth, and oregano, bring to a boil.

4. Reduce heat and simmer for 20 minutes.

5. Add cannellini beans and kale, cook for another 10 minutes. Season with salt and pepper. Serve hot.

Nutritional Facts (Per Serving): Calories: 600 | Carbs: 70g | Protein: 18g | Fat: 20g | Fiber: 16g | Sodium: 1100 mg | Sugars: 15g

CHAPTER 9: LUNCHES: Nutritious Grain and Legume Dishes

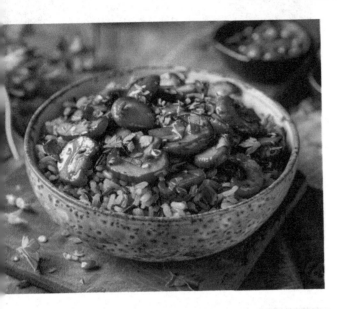

Mushroom and Wild Rice Pilaf

Prep: 10 minutes | Cook: 40 minutes | Serves: 2

Ingredients:

- 1 cup wild rice (180g)
- 2 cups vegetable broth (500ml)
- 1 tbsp olive oil (15ml)
- 1 cup mushrooms, sliced (90g)
- 1 small onion, finely chopped (70g)
- 1 clove garlic, minced
- 1/2 tsp salt (2.5g)
- 1/4 tsp black pepper (1g)
- 1/4 cup fresh parsley, chopped (15g)

Instructions:

1. Cook the wild rice in vegetable broth according to package instructions.
2. In a pan, heat olive oil over medium heat. Sauté onions and garlic until softened.
3. Add mushrooms, salt, and pepper, and cook until mushrooms are tender.
4. Stir in cooked wild rice and parsley. Mix well and heat through. Serve warm.

Nutritional Facts (Per Serving): Calories: 600 | Carbs: 90g | Protein: 14g | Fat: 18g | Fiber: 6g | Sodium: 800 mg | Sugars: 4g

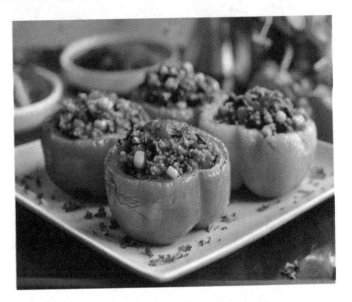

Quinoa and Black Bean Stuffed Peppers

Prep: 15 minutes | Cook: 35 minutes | Serves: 2

Ingredients:

- 2 large bell peppers (180g)
- 1/2 cup quinoa, rinsed (85g)
- 1 cup vegetable broth (250ml)
- 1 cup black beans, drained and rinsed (170g)
- 1/2 cup corn kernels, cherry tomatoes, halved (75g)
- 1 tsp cumin, paprika (2g each)
- 1/2 tsp salt (2.5g)
- 1/4 tsp black pepper (1g)
- 1/4 cup fresh cilantro, chopped (15g)
- 1/4 cup shredded cheese (30g)

Instructions:

1. Preheat oven to 375°F (190°C). Cut tops off bell peppers and remove seeds.
2. Cook quinoa in vegetable broth as directed.
3. Mix cooked quinoa, black beans, corn, tomatoes, cumin, paprika, salt, pepper, and cilantro in a bowl.
4. Stuff peppers with mixture, top with cheese.
5. Bake in a dish for 30-35 minutes until tender.

Nutritional Facts (Per Serving): Calories: 600 | Carbs: 85g | Protein: 18g | Fat: 18g | Fiber: 14g | Sodium: 900 mg | Sugars: 10g

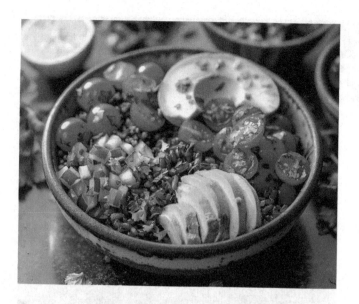

Red Rice and Avocado Bowl

Prep: 10 minutes | Cook: 30 minutes | Serves: 2

Ingredients:

- 1 cup red rice (180g)
- 2 cups water (500ml)
- 1 tbsp olive oil (15ml)
- 1 avocado, diced (150g)
- 1 cup cherry tomatoes, halved (150g)
- 1/4 cup red onion, finely chopped (40g)
- 1/4 cup fresh cilantro, chopped (15g)
- 1 lime, juiced (30g)
- 1/2 tsp salt (2.5g)
- 1/4 tsp black pepper (1g)

Instructions:

1. Cook red rice in water according to package instructions. Let it cool slightly.
2. In a bowl, combine cooked red rice, avocado, cherry tomatoes, red onion, and cilantro.
3. Drizzle with lime juice and olive oil. Season with salt and pepper.
4. Toss gently to combine.
5. Serve at room temperature.

Nutritional Facts (Per Serving): Calories: 600 | Carbs: 90g | Protein: 14g | Fat: 18g | Fiber: 6g | Sodium: 800 mg | Sugars: 4g

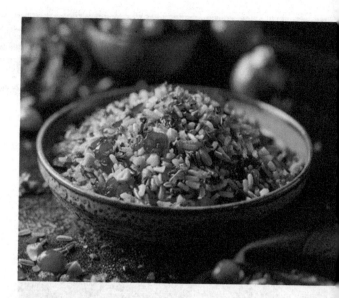

Wild Rice and Cranberry Pilaf

Prep: 10 minutes | Cook: 40 minutes | Serves: 2

Ingredients:

- 1 cup wild rice (180g)
- 2 cups vegetable broth (500ml)
- 1 tbsp olive oil (15ml)
- 1 small onion, finely chopped (70g)
- 1/2 cup dried cranberries (60g)
- 1/4 cup slivered almonds (30g)
- 1/2 tsp salt (2.5g)
- 1/4 tsp black pepper (1g)
- 1/4 cup fresh parsley, chopped (15g)

Instructions:

1. Cook wild rice in vegetable broth according to package instructions.
2. In a pan, heat olive oil over medium heat. Sauté onions until softened.
3. Stir in cooked wild rice, cranberries, almonds, salt, and pepper. Mix well and heat through.
4. Garnish with fresh parsley.
5. Serve warm.

Nutritional Facts (Per Serving): Calories: 600 | Carbs: 90g | Protein: 10g | Fat: 22g | Fiber: 8g | Sodium: 700 mg | Sugars: 18

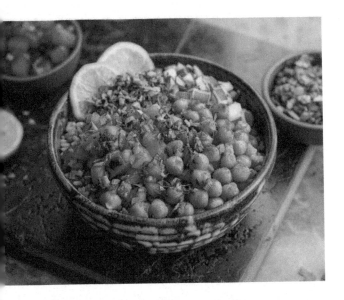

Spicy Chickpea and Brown Rice Bowl

Prep: 10 minutes | Cook: 20 minutes | Serves: 2

Ingredients:

- 1 cup brown rice (200g)
- 1 can chickpeas, drained and rinsed (400g)
- 1 tbsp olive oil (15ml)
- 1 tsp ground cumin, coriander (2g each)
- 1/2 tsp cayenne pepper (1g)
- 1/2 tsp salt (3g)
- 1 red bell pepper, diced (150g)
- 1/2 red onion, diced (75g)
- 1/4 cup fresh cilantro, chopped (10g)
- juice of 1 lime (30ml)

Instructions:

1. Cook the brown rice according to package instructions.
2. In a large pan, heat olive oil over medium heat.
3. Add chickpeas, cumin, coriander, cayenne pepper, and salt. Sauté for 5 minutes.
4. Add red bell pepper and red onion, cooking until softened, about 5 minutes.
5. Stir in cooked brown rice and cilantro. Squeeze lime juice over the mixture and toss to combine.
6. Serve warm.

Nutritional Facts (Per Serving): Calories: 600 | Carbs: 102g | Protein: 16g | Fat: 16g | Fiber: 16g | Sodium: 600 mg | Sugars: 5g

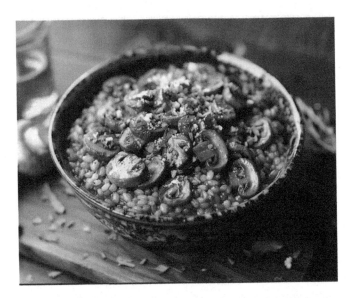

Barley and Mushroom Risotto

Prep: 10 minutes | Cook: 40 minutes | Serves: 2

Ingredients:

- 1 cup pearl barley (200g)
- 2 cups vegetable broth (500ml)
- 1 cup water (250ml)
- 1 tbsp olive oil (15ml)
- 1 small onion, finely chopped (100g)
- 2 garlic cloves, minced (6g)
- 1 cup mushrooms, sliced (100g)
- 1/2 cup Parmesan cheese, grated (50g)
- 1 tbsp butter (15g)
- 1/4 cup fresh parsley, chopped (10g)
- salt and pepper to taste

Instructions:

1. In a pot, bring vegetable broth and water to a simmer.
2. In a large pan, heat olive oil over medium heat. Add onion and garlic, cooking until softened, about 5 minutes.
3. Stir in barley and cook for 1 minute. Gradually add hot broth mixture, one ladle at a time, stirring constantly until absorbed before adding more.
4. Continue until barley is tender, about 30 minutes.
5. Stir in mushrooms in the last 10 minutes of cooking.
6. Remove from heat and stir in Parmesan cheese, butter, and parsley. Season with salt and pepper.
7. Serve warm.

Nutritional Facts (Per Serving): Calories: 600 | Carbs: 95g | Protein: 20g | Fat: 18g | Fiber: 12g | Sodium: 800 mg | Sugars: 6g

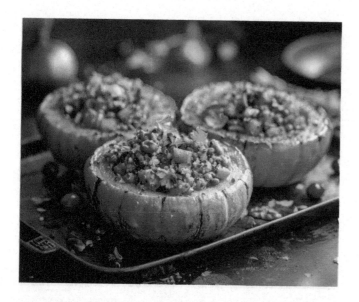

Green Lentil and Quinoa Stuffed Squash

Prep: 15 minutes | Cook: 45 minutes | Serves: 2

Ingredients:

- 2 acorn squashes, halved and seeded (800g total)
- 1 cup cooked green lentils (200g)
- 1/2 cup quinoa (85g)
- 1 cup vegetable broth (250ml)
- 1 small onion, finely chopped (100g)
- 1 garlic clove, minced (3g)
- 1 tbsp olive oil (15ml)
- 1/2 tsp ground cumin, cinnamon (2g each)
- 1/4 cup dried cranberries, chopped walnuts (30g each)
- Salt and pepper to taste

Instructions:

1. Preheat oven to 375 °F (190 °C). Place squash halves cut side down on a baking sheet and roast for 30 minutes.
2. In a saucepan, boil quinoa and vegetable broth. Reduce heat, cover, and simmer for 15 minutes.
3. In a pan, heat olive oil over medium heat. Add onion and garlic, cooking for 5 minutes. Stir in lentils, quinoa, cumin, cinnamon, cranberries, and walnuts. Season with salt and pepper.
4. Fill squash halves with the mixture. Bake for an additional 10 minutes. Serve warm.

Nutritional Facts (Per Serving): Calories: 600 | Carbs: 95g | Protein: 15g | Fat: 22g | Fiber: 15g | Sodium: 600 mg | Sugars: 12g

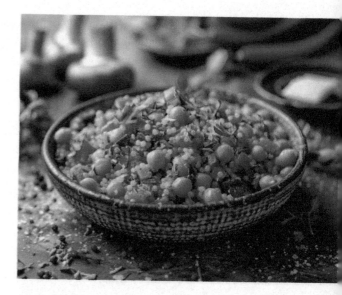

Couscous and Chickpea Pilaf

Prep: 10 minutes | Cook: 15 minutes | Serves: 2

Ingredients:

- 1 cup couscous (180g)
- 1 cup boiling water (250ml)
- 1 can chickpeas, drained and rinsed (400g)
- 1 tbsp olive oil (15ml)
- 1 small onion, finely chopped (100g)
- 1 carrot, grated (75g)
- 1/2 cup raisins (75g)
- 1/4 cup fresh parsley, chopped (10g)
- 1/2 tsp ground cumin (2g)
- 1/2 tsp ground turmeric (2g)
- salt and pepper to taste

Instructions:

1. Simmer vegetable broth and water in a pot.
2. Heat olive oil in a large pan over medium heat. Sauté onion and garlic for 5 minutes until softened.
3. Add barley and cook for 1 minute. Gradually add hot broth, stirring until absorbed before adding more.
4. Cook until barley is tender, about 30 minutes, adding mushrooms in the last 10 minutes.
5. Remove from heat and stir in Parmesan, butter, and parsley. Season with salt and pepper.
6. Serve warm.

Nutritional Facts (Per Serving): Calories: 600 | Carbs: 106g | Protein: 16g | Fat: 14g | Fiber: 13g | Sodium: 500 mg | Sugars: 15g

CHAPTER 10: LUNCHES: Quick and Easy One-Pot Meals

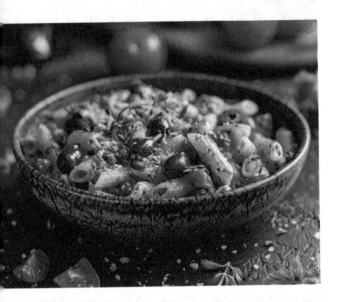

One-Pot Mediterranean Pasta with Olives

Prep: 10 minutes | Cook: 20 minutes | Serves: 2

Ingredients:

- 8 oz penne pasta (225g)
- 2 cups vegetable broth (500ml)
- 1 cup cherry tomatoes, halved (150g)
- 1/2 cup Kalamata olives, pitted and sliced (75g)
- 1/4 cup sun-dried tomatoes, chopped (40g)
- 1/4 cup feta cheese, crumbled (50g)
- 2 tbsp olive oil (30g)
- 1 tsp dried oregano (4g)
- 1/2 tsp salt, black pepper (1.5g, 0.6g)
- 2 cloves garlic, minced (8g)

Instructions:

1. In a large pot, heat olive oil over medium heat. Sauté garlic until fragrant.
2. Add pasta, vegetable broth, cherry tomatoes, olives, sun-dried tomatoes, oregano, salt, and pepper. Stir to combine.
3. Bring to a boil, then reduce heat and simmer, stirring occasionally, until pasta is cooked and liquid is absorbed, about 15-20 minutes.
4. Stir in crumbled feta cheese before serving.

Nutritional Facts (Per Serving): Calories: 600 | Carbs: 70g | Protein: 18g | Fat: 26g | Fiber: 5g | Sodium: 1400 mg | Sugars: 6g

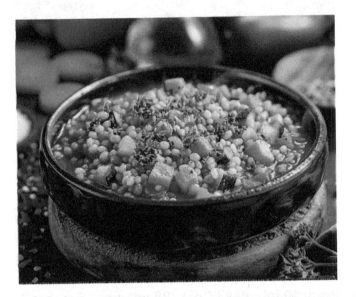

One-Pot Vegetable and Barley Casserole

Prep: 15 minutes | Cook: 45 minutes | Serves: 2

Ingredients:

- 1 cup pearl barley (200g)
- 2 cups vegetable broth (500ml)
- 1 cup celery, diced (100g)
- 1 cup bell pepper, zucchini, carrots, diced (150g each)
- 1/2 cup onion, chopped (75g)
- 2 tbsp olive oil (30g)
- 1 tsp dried thyme (4g)
- 1/2 tsp salt, black pepper (1.5g, 0.6g)

Instructions:

1. Heat olive oil in a large pot over medium heat. Sauté onion, carrots, celery, and bell pepper until softened, about 5 minutes.
2. Add barley, vegetable broth, zucchini, thyme, salt, and pepper. Stir well.
3. Bring to a boil, then reduce heat, cover, and simmer for 40-45 minutes, or until barley is tender and liquid is absorbed.

Nutritional Facts (Per Serving): Calories: 600 | Carbs: 94g | Protein: 12g | Fat: 16g | Fiber: 15g | Sodium: 800 mg | Sugars: 10g

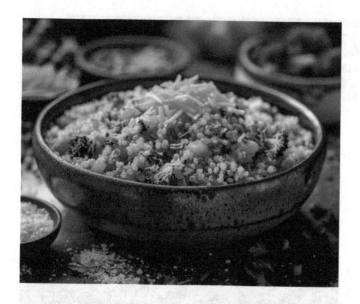

One-Pot Broccoli and Cheddar Quinoa

Prep: 10 minutes | Cook: 20 minutes | Serves: 2

Ingredients:

- 1 cup quinoa, rinsed (170g)
- 2 cups vegetable broth (500ml)
- 2 cups broccoli florets (150g)
- 1 cup shredded cheddar cheese (100g)
- 1/4 cup Parmesan cheese, grated (25g)
- 2 tbsp olive oil (30ml)
- 1/2 tsp salt (1.5g)
- 1/4 tsp black pepper, garlic powder (0.6g each)

Instructions:

1. In a large pot, heat olive oil over medium heat. Add quinoa and toast for 2 minutes.
2. Add vegetable broth, broccoli, salt, pepper, and garlic powder. Stir and bring to a boil.
3. Reduce heat, cover, and simmer for 15 minutes, or until quinoa is cooked and liquid is absorbed.
4. Stir in cheddar and Parmesan cheese until melted and well combined.

Nutritional Facts (Per Serving): Calories: 600 | Carbs: 50g | Protein: 28g | Fat: 32g | Fiber: 7g | Sodium: 1000 mg | Sugars: 4g

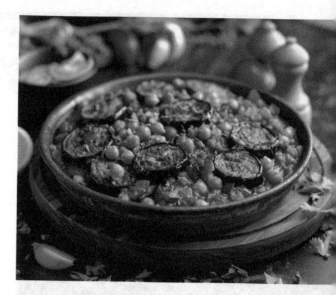

One-Pot Eggplant and Chickpea Tagine

Prep: 15 minutes | Cook: 30 minutes | Serves: 2

Ingredients:

- 1 medium eggplant, diced (250g)
- 1 can chickpeas, drained and rinsed (400g)
- 1 cup vegetable broth, crushed tomatoes (250ml each)
- 1/2 cup onion, chopped (75g)
- 2 cloves garlic, minced (8g)
- 2 tbsp olive oil (30ml)
- 1 tsp ground cumin, coriander (4g each)
- 1/2 tsp ground cinnamon
- 1/2 tsp cinnamon, salt, black pepper (1.5g, 0.6g)

Instructions:

1. Heat olive oil in a large pot over medium heat. Sauté onion and garlic until softened, about 3 minutes.
2. Add eggplant and cook until browned, about 5 minutes.
3. Stir in chickpeas, vegetable broth, crushed tomatoes, cumin, coriander, cinnamon, salt, and pepper. Bring to a boil.
4. Reduce heat, cover, and simmer for 20 minutes, stirring occasionally, until eggplant is tender.

Nutritional Facts (Per Serving): Calories: 600 | Carbs: 78g | Protein: 14g | Fat: 22g | Fiber: 18g | Sodium: 1000 mg | Sugars: 18g

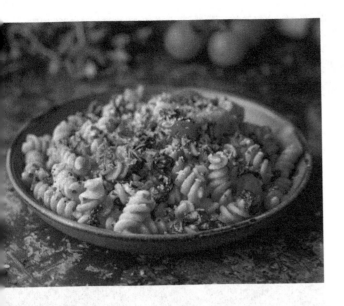

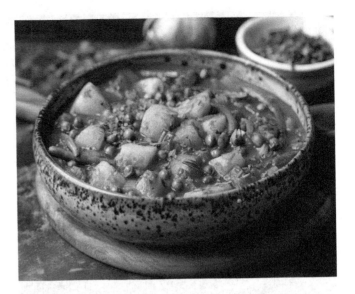

One-Pot Creamy Tomato and Spinach Pasta

Prep: 10 minutes | Cook: 20 minutes | Serves: 2

Ingredients:

- 8 oz fettuccine (225g)
- 2 cups vegetable broth (500ml)
- 1 cup crushed tomatoes (240ml)
- 1 cup fresh spinach, chopped (40g)
- 1/2 cup heavy cream (120ml)
- 1/4 cup Parmesan cheese, grated (25g)
- 2 tbsp olive oil (30ml)
- 2 cloves garlic, minced (8g)
- 1/2 tsp salt, black pepper (1.5g, 0.6g)

Instructions:

1. In a large pot, heat olive oil over medium heat. Sauté garlic until fragrant.
2. Add fettuccine, vegetable broth, crushed tomatoes, and salt. Stir to combine.
3. Bring to a boil, then reduce heat and simmer, stirring occasionally, until pasta is cooked and liquid is absorbed, about 15-20 minutes.
4. Stir in spinach, heavy cream, and Parmesan cheese until well combined.

Nutritional Facts (Per Serving): Calories: 600 | Carbs: 66g | Protein: 14g | Fat: 32g | Fiber: 4g | Sodium: 800 mg | Sugars: 8g

One-Pot Green Bean and Potato Stew

Prep: 15 minutes | Cook: 30 minutes | Serves: 2

Ingredients:

- 2 cups green beans, trimmed and cut into pieces (200g)
- 2 medium potatoes, diced (300g)
- 1 cup vegetable broth, crushed tomatoes (250ml each)
- 1/2 cup onion, chopped (75g)
- 2 cloves garlic, minced (8g)
- 2 tbsp olive oil (30ml)
- 1 tsp dried thyme (4g)
- 1/2 tsp salt, black pepper (1.5g, 0.6g)

Instructions:

1. Heat olive oil in a large pot over medium heat. Sauté onion and garlic until softened, about 3 minutes.
2. Add potatoes and cook for 5 minutes.
3. Stir in green beans, vegetable broth, crushed tomatoes, thyme, salt, and pepper. Bring to a boil.
4. Reduce heat, cover, and simmer for 20 minutes, or until potatoes are tender.

Nutritional Facts (Per Serving): Calories: 600 | Carbs: 80g | Protein: 8g | Fat: 28g | Fiber: 12g | Sodium: 800 mg | Sugars: 10g

CHAPTER 11: LUNCHES: Tasty Poultry and Meat Recipes

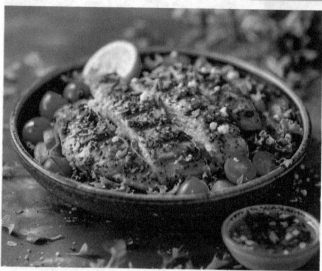

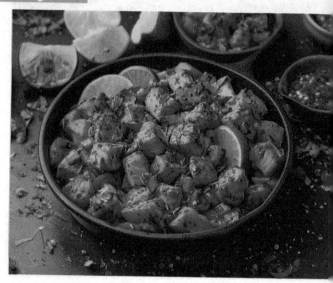

Lemon Herb Chicken and Quinoa Salad

Prep: 15 minutes | Cook: 20 minutes | Serves: 2

Ingredients:

- 2 boneless, skinless chicken breasts (about 300g)
- 1 cup cooked quinoa (185g)
- 2 cups mixed greens (60g)
- 1/2 cup cherry tomatoes, halved (75g)
- 1/4 cup red onion, thinly sliced (35g)
- 1/4 cup feta cheese, crumbled (50g)
- 2 tbsp olive oil (30ml)
- 2 tbsp lemon juice (30ml)
- 1 tsp dried oregano, garlic powder (2g each)
- salt and pepper to taste

Instructions:

1. Preheat grill to medium-high. Season chicken with oregano, garlic powder, salt, and pepper.
2. Grill chicken 6-7 minutes per side until cooked.
3. Let rest, then slice. In a large bowl, combine quinoa, greens, tomatoes, onion, and feta.
4. Whisk olive oil and lemon juice, drizzle over salad, toss to combine.
5. Top with sliced chicken and serve.

Nutritional Facts (Per Serving): Calories: 600 | Carbs: 30g | Protein: 45g | Fat: 30g | Fiber: 5g | Sodium: 700 mg | Sugars: 4g

Spicy Turkey and Sweet Potato Skillet

Prep: 10 minutes | Cook: 25 minutes | Serves: 2

Ingredients:

- 1 lb ground turkey (450g)
- 1 large sweet potato, diced (about 200g)
- 1 red bell pepper, diced (150g)
- 1/2 cup red onion, diced (75g)
- 2 cloves garlic, minced (8g)
- 1 tbsp olive oil (15ml)
- 1 tsp ground cumin, smoked paprika (2g each)
- 1/2 tsp cayenne pepper (1g)
- salt and pepper to taste
- 1/4 cup chopped cilantro (10g)

Instructions:

1. Heat olive oil in a large skillet over medium heat. Add garlic and onion, sauté for 2-3 minutes until fragrant.
2. Add ground turkey, cook until browned, about 5-7 minutes. Drain any excess fat.
3. Add sweet potato, red bell pepper, cumin, smoked paprika, cayenne pepper, salt, and pepper. Cook until sweet potatoes are tender, about 10-12 minutes.
4. Stir in chopped cilantro and serve.

Nutritional Facts (Per Serving): Calories: 600 | Carbs: 35g | Protein: 45g | Fat: 25g | Fiber: 7g | Sodium: 900 mg | Sugars: 10g

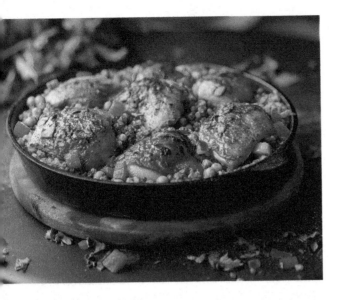

Herb-Roasted Chicken with Quinoa Pilaf

Prep: 10 minutes | Cook: 35 minutes | Serves: 2

Ingredients:

- 2 boneless, skinless chicken thighs (about 300g)
- 1 cup cooked quinoa (185g)
- 1/2 cup diced carrots, peas (75g each)
- 1/4 cup diced celery, onion (40g each)
- 2 tbsp olive oil (30ml)
- 1 tbsp chopped fresh parsley (10g)
- 1 tsp dried thyme (2g)
- salt and pepper to taste

Instructions:

1. Preheat oven to 375 °F (190 °C). Season chicken thighs with thyme, salt, and pepper. Heat 1 tbsp olive oil in an oven-safe skillet over medium-high heat.
2. Sear chicken thighs for 3-4 minutes per side until golden. Transfer skillet to oven and roast for 20-25 minutes until cooked.
3. In a separate pan, heat 1 tbsp olive oil. Sauté onion, carrots, celery, and peas for 5-7 minutes until tender. Stir in cooked quinoa and parsley. Season with salt and pepper.
4. Serve chicken thighs over quinoa pilaf.

Nutritional Facts (Per Serving): Calories: 600 | Carbs: 35g | Protein: 40g | Fat: 28g | Fiber: 6g | Sodium: 800 mg | Sugars: 5g

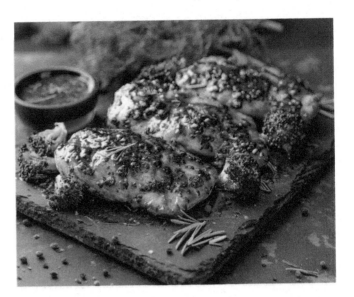

Honey Mustard Chicken and Broccoli

Prep: 10 minutes | Cook: 25 minutes | Serves: 2

Ingredients:

- 2 boneless, skinless chicken breasts (about 300g)
- 2 cups broccoli florets (150g)
- 2 tbsp olive oil, honey, Dijon mustard (30ml each)
- 1 tbsp whole grain mustard (15ml)
- 1 tsp garlic powder (2g)
- salt and pepper to taste

Instructions:

1. Preheat oven to 375 °F (190 °C). Mix honey, Dijon mustard, whole grain mustard, garlic powder, salt, and pepper in a small bowl.
2. Place chicken breasts in a baking dish and brush with the honey mustard mixture.
3. Toss broccoli with olive oil, salt, and pepper, and arrange around the chicken.
4. Bake for 25 minutes until chicken is cooked through and broccoli is tender.
5. Serve with any remaining sauce drizzled on top.

Nutritional Facts (Per Serving): Calories: 600 | Carbs: 30g | Protein: 45g | Fat: 25g | Fiber: 6g | Sodium: 600 mg | Sugars: 15g

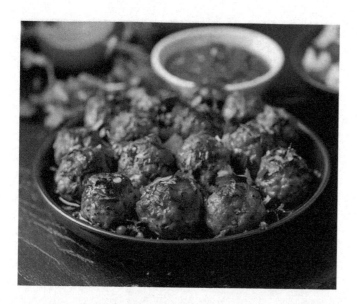

Moroccan Spiced Turkey Meatballs

Prep: 15 minutes | Cook: 20 minutes | Serves: 2

Ingredients:

- 1 lb ground turkey (450g)
- 1/2 cup almond flour (50g)
- 1 egg, beaten (50g)
- 1/4 cup finely chopped onion (35g)
- 2 cloves garlic, minced
- 2 tbsp chopped fresh cilantro (10g)
- 1 tbsp olive oil (15ml)
- 1 tsp ground cumin, coriander (2g each)
- 1/2 tsp ground cinnamon, paprika (1g each)
- salt and pepper to taste
- 1/2 cup Greek yogurt (125g)
- 1 tbsp lemon juice (15ml)

Instructions:

1. Preheat oven to 400 °F (200 °C). In a bowl, combine turkey, almond flour, egg, onion, garlic, cilantro, cumin, coriander, cinnamon, paprika, salt, and pepper. Mix well.

2. Form mixture into small meatballs and place on a baking sheet lined with parchment paper.

3. Drizzle meatballs with olive oil and bake for 18-20 minutes until fully cooked.

4. In a small bowl, mix Greek yogurt with lemon juice.

5. Serve meatballs with the yogurt sauce.

Nutritional Facts (Per Serving): Calories: 600 | Carbs: 15g | Protein: 50g | Fat: 35g | Fiber: 3g | Sodium: 700 mg | Sugars: 5g

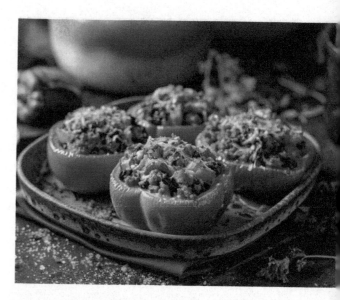

Chicken and Spinach Stuffed Peppers

Prep:15 minutes | Cook: 40 minutes | Serves: 2

Ingredients:

- 4 bell peppers, halved and seeded (4 large peppers)
- 1 lb ground chicken (450g)
- 2 cups fresh spinach, chopped (60g)
- 1 cup shredded mozzarella cheese (100g)
- 1 medium onion, diced (75g)
- 2 cloves garlic, minced (8g)
- 1 tsp dried oregano (4g)
- 1/2 tsp salt, black pepper (1.5g, 0.6g)
- 1 tbsp olive oil (15 ml)

Instructions:

1. Preheat oven to 375 °F (190 °C). Arrange pepper halves in a baking dish.

2. In a large pan, heat olive oil over medium heat. Sauté onion and garlic until soft.

3. Add ground chicken, cook until browned. Stir in spinach, oregano, salt, and pepper.

4. Fill each pepper half with the chicken mixture. Top with shredded mozzarella.

5. Bake for 30 minutes, until peppers are tender and cheese is melted and golden.

Nutritional Facts (Per Serving): Calories: 600 | Carbs: 10g | Protein: 45g | Fat: 35g | Fiber: 3g | Sodium: 900 mg | Sugars: 6g

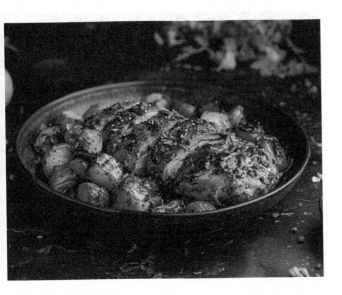

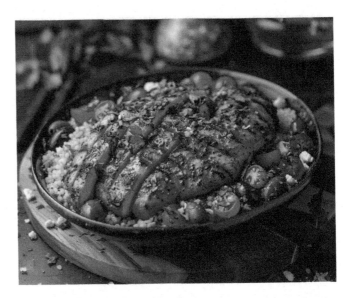

Balsamic Chicken and Roasted Vegetables

Mediterranean Chicken and Couscous

Prep 10 minutes | Cook: 30 minutes | Serves: 2

Prep: 10 minutes | Cook: 20 minutes | Serves: 2

Ingredients:

- 2 boneless, skinless chicken breasts (2 large breasts)
- 1/4 cup balsamic vinegar (60 ml)
- 2 tbsp olive oil (30 ml)
- 2 cups broccoli florets (150g)
- 1 red bell pepper, zucchini, sliced (75 each)
- 1 tsp dried thyme (4g)
- 1/2 tsp salt, black pepper (1.5g, 0.6g)

Ingredients:

- 2 boneless, skinless chicken breasts (2 large breasts)
- 1 cup couscous (180g)
- 1 cup chicken broth (240 ml)
- 1/2 cup cherry tomatoes, halved (75g)
- 1/4 cup Kalamata olives, pitted and sliced (40g)
- 1/4 cup feta cheese, crumbled (40g)
- 1 tbsp olive oil (15 ml)
- 1 tsp dried oregano (4g)
- 1/2 tsp salt, black pepper (1.5g, 0.6g)

Instructions:

1. Preheat oven to 400 °F (200 °C). Line a baking sheet with parchment paper.
2. In a bowl, mix balsamic vinegar, olive oil, thyme, salt, and pepper. Marinate chicken in this mixture for 10 minutes.
3. Arrange chicken and vegetables on the baking sheet. Drizzle remaining marinade over vegetables.
4. Roast for 25-30 minutes, until chicken is cooked through and vegetables are tender.

Instructions:

1. Cook couscous according to package instructions using chicken broth.
2. In a pan, heat olive oil over medium heat. Season chicken with oregano, salt, and pepper. Cook until golden and cooked through.
3. Slice chicken and arrange over cooked couscous.
4. Top with cherry tomatoes, olives, and feta.

Nutritional Facts (Per Serving): Calories: 600 | Carbs: 15g | Protein: 45g | Fat: 35g | Fiber: 5g | Sodium: 800 mg | Sugars: 10g

Nutritional Facts (Per Serving): Calories: 600 | Carbs: 45g | Protein: 40g | Fat: 25g | Fiber: 5g | Sodium: 1000 mg | Sugars: 5g

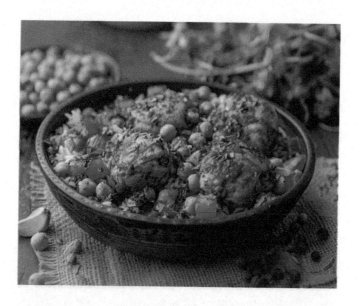

Chicken and Chickpea Tagine

Prep: 15 minutes | Cook: 40 minutes | Serves: 2

Ingredients:

- 2 boneless, skinless chicken thighs (2 large thighs)
- 1 cup canned chickpeas, drained and rinsed (165g)
- 1 cup diced tomatoes (240 ml)
- 1 medium onion, diced (75g)
- 2 cloves garlic, minced (8g)
- 1 tsp ground cumin, coriander, cinnamon (2g each)
- 1/2 tsp salt, black pepper (1.5g, 0.6g)
- 1 tbsp olive oil (15 ml)
- 1 cup chicken broth (240 ml)

Instructions:

1. Heat olive oil in a large pot over medium heat. Sauté onion and garlic until soft.
2. Add chicken, cook until browned. Stir in spices and cook for 1 minute.
3. Add chickpeas, tomatoes, and chicken broth. Simmer for 30 minutes until chicken is tender and sauce thickens.

Nutritional Facts (Per Serving): Calories: 600 | Carbs: 30g | Protein: 40g | Fat: 30g | Fiber: 8g | Sodium: 900 mg | Sugars: 8g

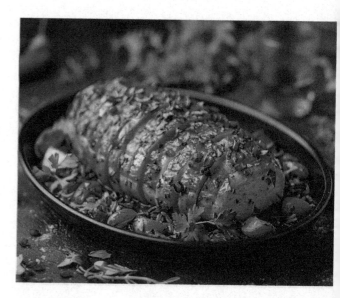

Herb-Crusted Turkey and Wild Rice

Prep: 15 minutes | Cook: 40 minutes | Serves:2

Ingredients:

- 2 turkey tenderloins (2 large tenderloins)
- 1/2 cup wild rice (90g)
- 1 cup chicken broth (240 ml)
- 1 tbsp olive oil (15 ml)
- 1 tbsp fresh parsley, thyme, chopped (15g)
- 1 tsp dried rosemary (2g)
- 1/2 tsp salt, black pepper (1.5g, 0.6g)

Instructions:

1. Preheat oven to 375 °F (190 °C). Rub turkey with olive oil, parsley, thyme, rosemary, salt, and pepper.
2. Cook wild rice according to package instructions using chicken broth.
3. Place turkey in a baking dish and roast for 25-30 minutes until cooked through.
4. Serve turkey slices over wild rice.

Nutritional Facts (Per Serving): Calories: 600 | Carbs: 25g | Protein: 45g | Fat: 30g | Fiber: 4g | Sodium: 800 mg | Sugars: 2g

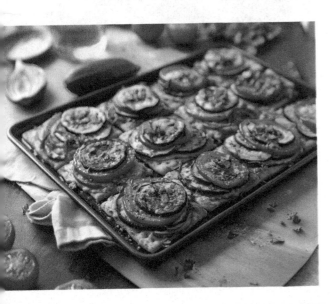

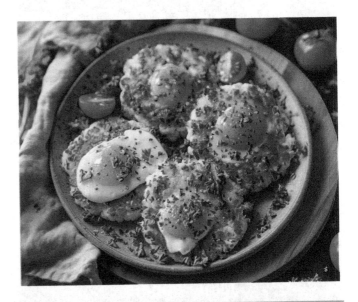

Roasted Veggie and Hummus Flatbread

Prep: 15 minutes | Cook: 25 minutes | Serves: 4

Ingredients:

- 2 cups cherry tomatoes, halved (300g)
- 1 medium zucchini, sliced (200g)
- 1 red bell pepper, sliced (150g)
- 2 tbsp olive oil (30ml)
- Salt and pepper to taste
- 4 whole wheat flatbreads (300g total)
- 1 cup hummus (240g)
- 1 tsp dried oregano (5g)
- 2 cups mixed greens (100g)

Instructions:

1. Preheat oven to 400°F (200°C).
2. Toss cherry tomatoes, zucchini, and red bell pepper with olive oil, salt, and pepper. Spread on a baking sheet.
3. Roast vegetables for 20-25 minutes until tender and slightly caramelized.
4. Warm flatbreads in the oven for 5 minutes.
5. Spread hummus evenly on each flatbread. Top with roasted vegetables and sprinkle with oregano.
6. Garnish with mixed greens before serving.

Nutritional Facts (Per Serving): Calories: 400 | Sugars: 6g | Fat: 18g | Carbohydrates: 50g | Protein: 12g | Fiber: 8g | Sodium: 400mg

Cauliflower Hash Browns with Poached Eggs

Prep: 15 minutes | Cook: 20 minutes | Serves: 4

Ingredients:

- 4 cups grated cauliflower (500g)
- 1/2 cup shredded cheddar cheese (60g)
- 1/4 cup almond flour (30g)
- 2 eggs, beaten (100g)
- Salt and pepper to taste
- 1 tbsp olive oil (15ml)
- 4 large eggs, poached
- 1 tbsp chopped chives (5g)

Instructions:

1. In a large bowl, combine grated cauliflower, cheddar cheese, almond flour, beaten eggs, salt, and pepper.
2. Heat olive oil in a large skillet over medium heat.
3. Form cauliflower mixture into patties and cook for 4-5 minutes on each side until golden brown.
4. Poach the eggs in simmering water for 3-4 minutes until whites are set but yolks remain runny.
5. Serve hash browns topped with poached eggs and garnished with chives.

Nutritional Facts (Per Serving): Calories: 400 | Sugars: 3g | Fat: 28g | Carbohydrates: 12g | Protein: 23g | Fiber: 5g | Sodium: 500mg

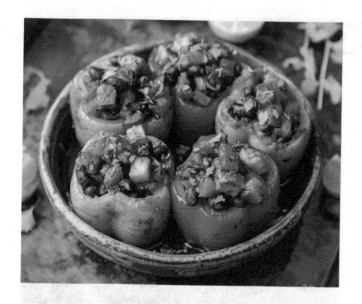

Avocado and Black Bean Stuffed Mini Peppers

Prep: 10 minutes | Cook: 10 minutes | Serves: 4

Ingredients:

- 1 lb mini bell peppers, halved and seeded (450g)
- 1 can black beans, rinsed and drained (240g)
- 1 large avocado, diced (200g)
- 1/2 cup diced red onion (60g)
- 1/4 cup chopped cilantro (15g)
- 1 tbsp lime juice (15ml)
- Salt and pepper to taste
- 1 tbsp olive oil (15ml)

Instructions:

1. Preheat oven to 375°F (190°C).
2. Place mini bell peppers on a baking sheet and drizzle with olive oil. Roast for 10 minutes until tender.
3. In a medium bowl, combine black beans, avocado, red onion, cilantro, lime juice, salt, and pepper.
4. Stuff each mini bell pepper half with the avocado and black bean mixture.
5. Serve immediately.

Nutritional Facts (Per Serving): Calories: 400 | Sugars: 5g | Fat: 22g | Carbohydrates: 45g | Protein: 10g | Fiber: 15g | Sodium: 300mg

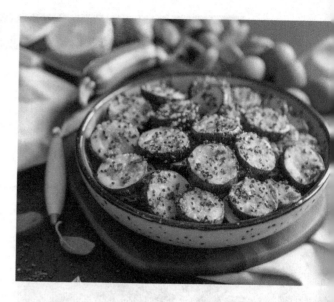

Zucchini and Quinoa Bites

Prep: 15 minutes | Cook: 20 minutes | Serves: 4

Ingredients:

- 1 cup cooked quinoa (170g)
- 2 medium zucchinis, grated (300g)
- 1/2 cup grated Parmesan cheese (50g)
- 2 eggs, beaten (100g)
- 1/4 cup almond flour (30g)
- 1 tsp garlic powder (5g)
- Salt and pepper to taste
- 1 tbsp olive oil (15ml)

Instructions:

1. Preheat oven to 375°F (190°C).
2. In a large bowl, combine cooked quinoa, grated zucchinis, Parmesan cheese, beaten eggs, almond flour, garlic powder, salt, and pepper.
3. Form mixture into small balls and place on a baking sheet lined with parchment paper.
4. Brush with olive oil and bake for 15-20 minutes until golden brown.
5. Serve warm.

Nutritional Facts (Per Serving): Calories: 400 Sugars: 3g | Fat: 22g | Carbohydrates: 32g Protein: 15g | Fiber: 5g | Sodium: 300mg

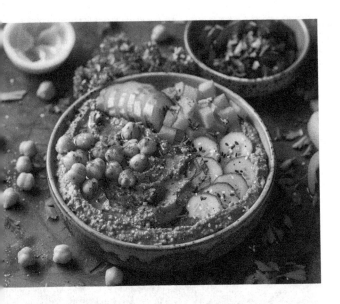

Beet and Walnut Hummus with Crudités

Prep: 10 minutes | Cook: 45 minutes | Serves: 4

Ingredients:

- 2 medium beets, roasted and peeled (300g)
- 1 can chickpeas, drained and rinsed (240g)
- 1/4 cup walnuts (30g)
- 2 tbsp tahini (30g)
- 2 tbsp lemon juice (30ml)
- 2 tbsp olive oil (30ml)
- 1 garlic clove (5g)
- Salt and pepper to taste
- Assorted crudités (carrots, cucumbers, bell peppers) (400g)

Instructions:

1. Preheat oven to 400°F (200°C). Wrap beets in foil and roast for 45 minutes until tender. Let cool and peel.
2. In a food processor, combine roasted beets, chickpeas, walnuts, tahini, lemon juice, olive oil, garlic, salt, and pepper. Blend until smooth.
3. Serve hummus with assorted crudités.

Nutritional Facts (Per Serving): Calories: 400 | Sugars: 8g | Fat: 24g | Carbohydrates: 38g | Protein: 10g | Fiber: 10g | Sodium: 200mg

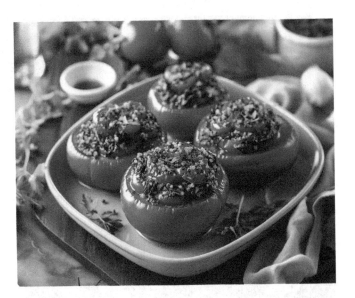

Quinoa and Spinach Stuffed Tomatoes

Prep: 15 minutes | Cook: 30 minutes | Serves: 4

Ingredients:

- 4 large tomatoes (600g)
- 1 cup cooked quinoa (170g)
- 2 cups fresh spinach, chopped (60g)
- 1/4 cup feta cheese, crumbled (40g)
- 1 small onion, finely chopped (70g)
- 2 garlic cloves, minced (10g)
- 1 tbsp olive oil (15ml)
- Salt and pepper to taste

Instructions:

1. Preheat oven to 375°F (190°C).
2. Slice tops off tomatoes and scoop out the insides. Set aside.
3. In a skillet, heat olive oil over medium heat. Sauté onion and garlic until softened, about 5 minutes.
4. Add spinach and cook until wilted. Stir in cooked quinoa and feta cheese, and season with salt and pepper.
5. Stuff tomatoes with quinoa mixture and place in a baking dish. Bake for 25-30 minutes until tomatoes are tender.

Nutritional Facts (Per Serving): Calories: 400 | Sugars: 10g | Fat: 18g | Carbohydrates: 45g | Protein: 12g | Fiber: 8g | Sodium: 350mg

CHAPTER 13: SNACKS: Appetizing Dips and Spreads

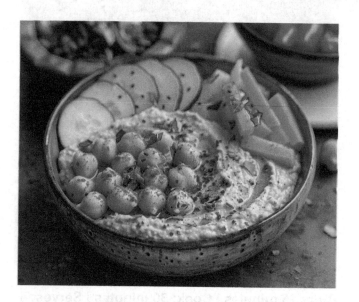

Classic Hummus with Paprika

Prep: 10 minutes | Serves: 4

Ingredients:

- 1 can chickpeas, drained and rinsed (240g)
- 1/4 cup tahini (60g)
- 2 tbsp lemon juice (30ml)
- 2 tbsp olive oil (30ml)
- 1 garlic clove (5g)
- 1 tsp ground cumin (5g)
- 1/2 tsp sea salt (2.5g)
- 1/2 tsp smoked paprika (2.5g)
- 2-3 tbsp water (30-45ml)

Instructions:

1. In a food processor, combine chickpeas, tahini, lemon juice, olive oil, garlic, cumin, and sea salt.
2. Blend until smooth, adding water as needed to reach desired consistency.
3. Transfer to a serving bowl and sprinkle with smoked paprika.
4. Serve with pita bread or vegetable sticks.

Nutritional Facts (Per Serving): Calories: 400 | Sugars: 1g | Fat: 22g | Carbohydrates: 36g | Protein: 12g | Fiber: 10g | Sodium: 450mg

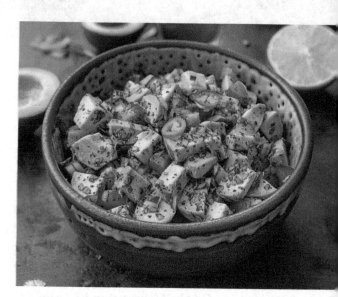

Avocado and Cilantro Salsa

Prep: 10 minutes | Serves: 4

Ingredients:

- 2 large avocados, diced (400g)
- 1 cup cherry tomatoes, quartered (150g)
- 1/4 cup red onion, finely chopped (40g)
- 1/4 cup fresh cilantro, chopped (15g)
- 1 tbsp lime juice (15ml)
- 1 tbsp olive oil (15ml)
- 1/2 tsp sea salt (2.5g)
- 1/2 tsp black pepper (2.5g)

Instructions:

1. In a medium bowl, combine diced avocados, cherry tomatoes, red onion, and fresh cilantro.
2. Drizzle with lime juice and olive oil.
3. Season with sea salt and black pepper.
4. Gently toss to combine.
5. Serve immediately with tortilla chips or as a topping for grilled fish or chicken.

Nutritional Facts (Per Serving): Calories: 400 | Sugars: 3g | Fat: 33g | Carbohydrates: 27g | Protein: 5g | Fiber: 12g | Sodium: 300mg

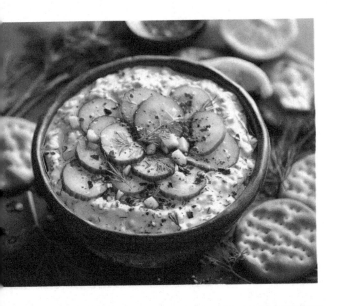

Cucumber and Dill Greek Yogurt Dip

Prep: 10 minutes | Serves: 4

Ingredients:

- 2 cups Greek yogurt (480g)
- 1 large cucumber, grated and drained (300g)
- 2 tbsp fresh dill, chopped (10g)
- 1 garlic clove, minced (5g)
- 1 tbsp lemon juice (15ml)
- 1 tbsp olive oil (15ml)
- 1/2 tsp sea salt (2.5g)
- 1/4 tsp black pepper (1.25g)

Instructions:

1. In a medium bowl, combine Greek yogurt, grated cucumber, fresh dill, garlic, lemon juice, olive oil, sea salt, and black pepper.
2. Mix well until all ingredients are evenly distributed.
3. Serve chilled with pita bread or vegetable sticks.

Nutritional Facts (Per Serving): Calories: 400 | Sugars: 10g | Fat: 22g | Carbohydrates: 25g | Protein: 24g | Fiber: 2g | Sodium: 300mg

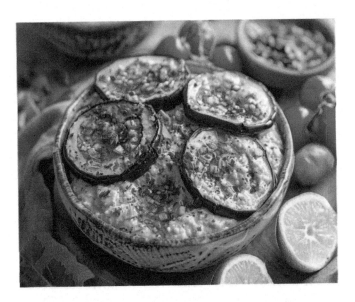

Smoky Eggplant Baba Ganoush

Prep: 10 minutes | Cook: 40 minutes | Serves: 4

Ingredients:

- 2 large eggplants (600g)
- 1/4 cup tahini (60g)
- 2 tbsp olive oil (30ml)
- 2 tbsp lemon juice (30ml)
- 2 garlic cloves, minced (10g)
- 1/2 tsp smoked paprika (2.5g)
- 1/2 tsp sea salt (2.5g)
- 1/4 tsp black pepper (1.25g)

Instructions:

1. Preheat oven to 400°F (200°C). Prick eggplants with a fork and roast on a baking sheet for 35-40 minutes until tender.
2. Let eggplants cool, then scoop out the flesh and place it in a food processor.
3. Add tahini, olive oil, lemon juice, garlic, smoked paprika, sea salt, and black pepper to the food processor.
4. Blend until smooth and creamy.
5. Serve with warm pita bread or vegetable sticks.

Nutritional Facts (Per Serving): Calories: 400 | Sugars: 8g | Fat: 28g | Carbohydrates: 34g | Protein: 6g | Fiber: 14g | Sodium: 300mg

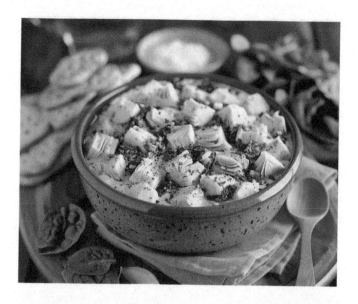

Artichoke and Spinach Yogurt Dip

Prep: 10 minutes | Cook: 10 minutes | Serves: 4

Ingredients:

- 1 cup plain Greek yogurt (240g)
- 1 cup canned artichoke hearts, drained and chopped (240g)
- 2 cups fresh spinach, chopped (60g)
- 1/4 cup grated Parmesan cheese (25g)
- 1 garlic clove, minced (5g)
- 1 tbsp lemon juice (15ml)
- 1 tbsp olive oil (15ml)
- 1/2 tsp sea salt (2.5g)
- 1/4 tsp black pepper (1.25g)

Instructions:

1. In a skillet, heat olive oil over medium heat. Sauté spinach and garlic until wilted, about 3 minutes.

2. In a bowl, combine Greek yogurt, chopped artichoke hearts, sautéed spinach, Parmesan cheese, lemon juice, sea salt, and black pepper. Mix well.

3. Serve with whole grain crackers or vegetable sticks.

Nutritional Facts (Per Serving): Calories: 400 | Sugars: 4g | Fat: 22g | Carbohydrates: 30g | Protein: 18g | Fiber: 6g | Sodium: 500mg

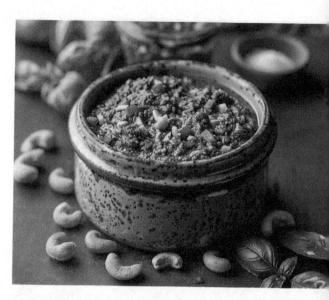

Cashew and Herb Pesto

Prep: 10 minutes | Serves: 4

Ingredients:

- 1 cup raw cashews (140g)
- 2 cups fresh basil leaves (50g)
- 1/2 cup fresh parsley (30g)
- 1/2 cup grated Parmesan cheese (50g)
- 1/4 cup olive oil (60ml)
- 2 garlic cloves (10g)
- 1 tbsp lemon juice (15ml)
- 1/2 tsp sea salt (2.5g)
- 1/4 tsp black pepper (1.2

Instructions:

1. In a food processor, combine cashews, basil leaves, parsley, Parmesan cheese, garlic, lemon juice, sea salt, and black pepper.

2. With the processor running, slowly add olive oil until the mixture is smooth and well combined.

3. Serve as a dip, spread, or pasta sauce.

Nutritional Facts (Per Serving): Calories: 400 Sugars: 3g | Fat: 34g | Carbohydrates: 18g Protein: 10g | Fiber: 4g | Sodium: 400mg

CHAPTER 14: SNACKS: Healthy Finger Foods

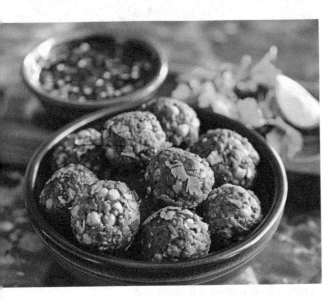

Baked Falafel Balls

Prep: 15 minutes | Cook: 25 minutes | Serves: 4

Ingredients:

- 1 can chickpeas, drained and rinsed (240g)
- 1/2 cup chopped onion (75g)
- 1/4 cup fresh parsley (15g)
- 1/4 cup fresh cilantro (15g)
- 2 garlic cloves (10g)
- 2 tbsp lemon juice (30ml)
- 2 tbsp olive oil (30ml)
- 1 tsp ground cumin (5g)
- 1 tsp ground coriander (5g)
- 1/2 tsp baking powder (2.5g)
- 1/2 tsp sea salt (2.5g)
- 1/4 tsp black pepper (1.25g)

Instructions:

1. Preheat oven to 375°F (190°C).
2. In a food processor, combine chickpeas, onion, parsley, cilantro, garlic, lemon juice, olive oil, cumin, coriander, baking powder, sea salt, and black pepper. Blend until smooth.
3. Form mixture into small balls and place on a baking sheet lined with parchment paper.
4. Bake for 20-25 minutes until golden brown.
5. Serve with tahini sauce or a green salad.

Nutritional Facts (Per Serving): Calories: 400 | Sugars: 2g | Fat: 18g | Carbohydrates: 48g | Protein: 10g | Fiber: 12g | Sodium: 450mg

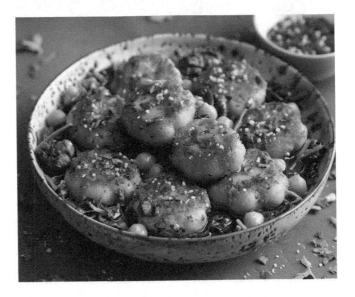

Chickpea and Spinach Patties

Prep: 15 minutes | Cook: 20 minutes | Serves: 4

Ingredients:

- 1 can chickpeas, drained and rinsed (240g)
- 2 cups fresh spinach, chopped (60g)
- 1/2 cup chopped onion (75g)
- 2 garlic cloves, minced (10g)
- 1/4 cup whole wheat flour (30g)
- 1 egg (50g)
- 1 tbsp lemon juice (15ml)
- 1 tsp ground cumin (5g)
- 1 tsp ground coriander (5g)
- Salt and pepper to taste
- 2 tbsp olive oil (30ml)

Instructions:

1. In a food processor, combine chickpeas, spinach, onion, garlic, whole wheat flour, egg, lemon juice, cumin, coriander, salt, and pepper. Pulse until well mixed but still slightly chunky.
2. Form the mixture into small patties.
3. Heat olive oil in a skillet over medium heat. Cook patties for 4-5 minutes on each side until golden brown.

Nutritional Facts (Per Serving): Calories: 400 | Sugars: 2g | Fat: 18g | Carbohydrates: 48g | Protein: 12g | Fiber: 12g | Sodium: 400mg

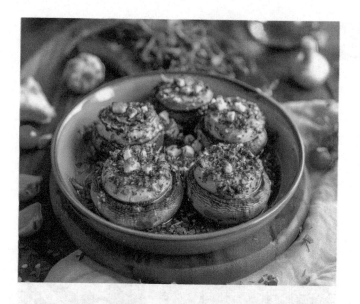

Zucchini and Feta Stuffed Mushrooms

Prep: 10 minutes | Cook: 20 minutes | Serves: 4

Ingredients:

- 12 large mushrooms, stems removed (300g)
- 1 medium zucchini, grated (200g)
- 1/2 cup crumbled feta cheese (75g)
- 1/4 cup breadcrumbs (30g)
- 2 garlic cloves, minced (10g)
- 1 tbsp olive oil (15ml)
- 1 tbsp fresh parsley, chopped (5g)
- Salt and pepper to taste

Instructions:

1. Preheat oven to 375°F (190°C).
2. In a bowl, combine grated zucchini, feta cheese, breadcrumbs, garlic, olive oil, parsley, salt, and pepper.
3. Stuff mushroom caps with the zucchini mixture and place on a baking sheet.
4. Bake for 15-20 minutes until mushrooms are tender and the filling is golden brown.
5. Serve warm.

Nutritional Facts (Per Serving): Calories: 400 | Sugars: 5g | Fat: 25g | Carbohydrates: 30g | Protein: 12g | Fiber: 8g | Sodium: 500mg

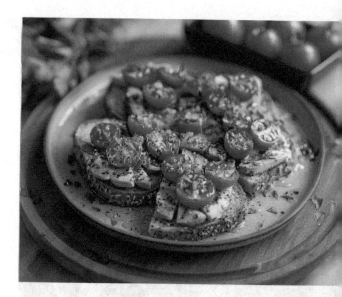

Mini Avocado Toasts with Tomato

Prep: 10 minutes | Serves: 4

Ingredients:

- 4 slices whole grain bread, toasted (200g)
- 2 large avocados, mashed (400g)
- 1 cup cherry tomatoes, halved (150g)
- 1 tbsp lemon juice (15ml)
- 1 tbsp olive oil (15ml)
- Salt and pepper to taste
- 1 tbsp fresh basil, chopped (5g)

Instructions:

1. In a bowl, mash avocados with lemon juice, olive oil, salt, and pepper.
2. Spread mashed avocado evenly over toasted bread slices.
3. Top with halved cherry tomatoes and sprinkle with chopped basil.
4. Serve immediately.

Nutritional Facts (Per Serving): Calories: 400 | Sugars: 5g | Fat: 28g | Carbohydrates: 36g | Protein: 8g | Fiber: 14g | Sodium: 300mg

CHAPTER 15: DESSERTS: Sweet and Savory Bites

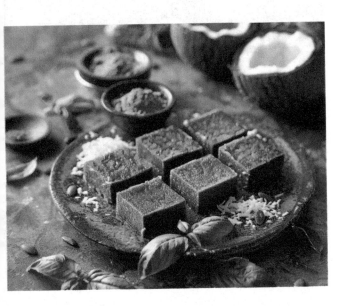

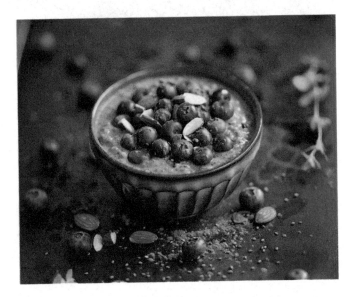

Coconut and Matcha Energy Bars

Prep: 15 minutes | Serves: 8

Ingredients:

- 2 cups shredded coconut (160g)
- 1 cup almond flour (120g)
- 1/2 cup coconut oil, melted (120ml)
- 1/4 cup honey or low carb sweetener (60ml)
- 1 tbsp matcha powder (15g)
- 1 tsp vanilla extract (5ml)
- Pinch of salt

Instructions:

1. In a large bowl, combine shredded coconut, almond flour, melted coconut oil, honey, matcha powder, vanilla extract, and a pinch of salt.
2. Mix well until all ingredients are fully combined.
3. Press the mixture firmly into an 8x8 inch (20x20cm) baking dish lined with parchment paper.
4. Refrigerate for at least 2 hours until set.
5. Cut into bars and serve.

Nutritional Facts (Per Serving): Calories: 400 | Sugars: 8g | Fat: 38g | Carbohydrates: 15g | Protein: 5g | Fiber: 6g | Sodium: 60mg

Chia Seed Pudding with Almonds and Blueberries

Prep: 10 minutes | Serves: 4

Ingredients:

- 2 cups almond milk (480ml)
- 1/2 cup chia seeds (80g)
- 1/4 cup honey or low carb sweetener (60ml)
- 1 tsp vanilla extract (5ml)
- 1/2 cup sliced almonds (60g)
- 1 cup fresh blueberries (150g)

Instructions:

1. In a medium bowl, whisk together almond milk, chia seeds, honey, and vanilla extract.
2. Let the mixture sit for 10 minutes, then whisk again to prevent clumping.
3. Cover and refrigerate for at least 4 hours or overnight until the pudding thickens.
4. Serve topped with sliced almonds and fresh blueberries.

Nutritional Facts (Per Serving): Calories: 400 | Sugars: 15g | Fat: 22g | Carbohydrates: 39g | Protein: 9g | Fiber: 15g | Sodium: 150mg

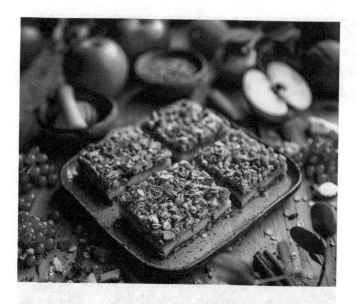

Apple and Cinnamon Oat Bars

Prep: 15 minutes | Cook: 25 minutes | Serves: 8

Ingredients:

- 2 cups rolled oats (180g)
- 1 cup unsweetened applesauce (240g)
- 1/2 cup almond butter (120g)
- 1/4 cup honey or low carb sweetener (60ml)
- 1/4 cup chopped walnuts (30g)
- 1 tsp ground cinnamon (5g)
- 1/2 tsp vanilla extract (2.5ml)
- Pinch of salt

Instructions:

1. Preheat oven to 350°F (175°C).
2. In a large bowl, combine rolled oats, applesauce, almond butter, honey, chopped walnuts, ground cinnamon, vanilla extract, and a pinch of salt.
3. Mix well until all ingredients are fully combined.
4. Press the mixture firmly into an 8x8 inch (20x20cm) baking dish lined with parchment paper.
5. Bake for 20-25 minutes until golden brown.
6. Let cool completely before cutting into bars.

Nutritional Facts (Per Serving): Calories: 400 | Sugars: 15g | Fat: 18g | Carbohydrates: 50g | Protein: 8g | Fiber: 6g | Sodium: 100mg

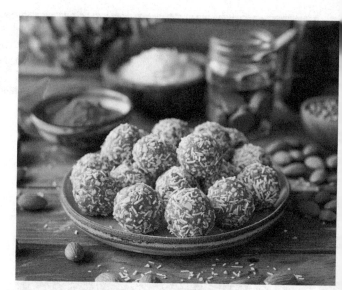

Ginger and Turmeric Bliss Balls

Prep: 15 minutes | Serves: 8

Ingredients:

- 1 cup almonds (150g)
- 1 cup medjool dates, pitted (200g)
- 1/4 cup unsweetened shredded coconut (30g)
- 1 tbsp fresh ginger, grated (15g)
- 1 tsp ground turmeric (5g)
- 1 tbsp coconut oil (15ml)
- 1 tsp vanilla extract (5ml)
- Pinch of salt

Instructions:

1. In a food processor, blend almonds until finely ground.
2. Add dates, shredded coconut, grated ginger, ground turmeric, coconut oil, vanilla extract, and a pinch of salt. Process until the mixture comes together.
3. Roll mixture into small balls and refrigerate for at least 1 hour until firm.
4. Serve chilled.

Nutritional Facts (Per Serving): Calories: 400 | Sugars: 22g | Fat: 24g | Carbohydrates: 38g | Protein: 8g | Fiber: 8g | Sodium: 30mg

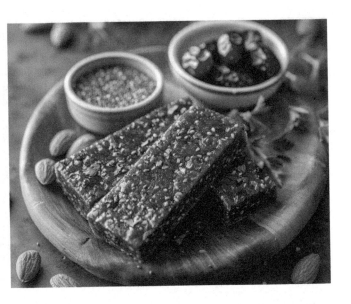

Almond Butter and Date Bars

Prep: 15 minutes | Serves: 8

Ingredients:

- 1 cup almond butter (240g)
- 1 cup medjool dates, pitted (200g)
- 1/2 cup rolled oats (45g)
- 1/4 cup chia seeds (40g)
- 1 tbsp coconut oil (15ml)
- 1 tsp vanilla extract (5ml)
- Pinch of salt

Instructions:

1. In a food processor, combine almond butter, dates, rolled oats, chia seeds, coconut oil, vanilla extract, and a pinch of salt. Process until smooth.
2. Press the mixture into an 8x8 inch (20x20cm) baking dish lined with parchment paper.
3. Refrigerate for at least 2 hours until firm.
4. Cut into bars and serve.

Nutritional Facts (Per Serving): Calories: 400 | Sugars: 24g | Fat: 24g | Carbohydrates: 40g | Protein: 10g | Fiber: 10g | Sodium: 50mg

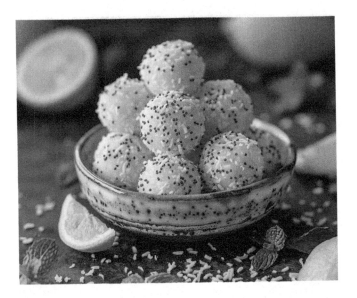

Lemon and Poppy Seed Energy Balls

Prep: 15 minutes | Serves: 8

Ingredients:

- 1 cup cashews (150g)
- 1 cup medjool dates, pitted (200g)
- 1/4 cup poppy seeds (30g)
- 2 tbsp lemon juice (30ml)
- Zest of 1 lemon (5g)
- 1 tbsp coconut oil (15ml)
- 1 tsp vanilla extract (5ml)
- Pinch of salt

Instructions:

1. In a food processor, blend cashews until finely ground.
2. Add dates, poppy seeds, lemon juice, lemon zest, coconut oil, vanilla extract, and a pinch of salt. Process until the mixture comes together.
3. Roll mixture into small balls and refrigerate for at least 1 hour until firm.
4. Serve chilled.

Nutritional Facts (Per Serving): Calories: 400 | Sugars: 22g | Fat: 22g | Carbohydrates: 44g | Protein: 8g | Fiber: 8g | Sodium: 30mg

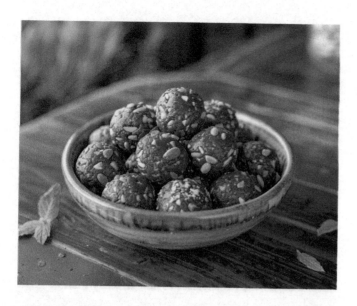

Cacao and Almond Protein Bites

Prep: 15 minutes | Serves: 8

Ingredients:

- 1 cup almonds (150g)
- 1 cup medjool dates, pitted (200g)
- 1/4 cup cacao powder (30g)
- 1/4 cup almond butter (60g)
- 2 tbsp protein powder (30g)
- 1 tbsp coconut oil (15ml)
- 1 tsp vanilla extract (5ml)
- Pinch of salt

Instructions:

1. In a food processor, blend almonds until finely ground.
2. Add dates, cacao powder, almond butter, protein powder, coconut oil, vanilla extract, and a pinch of salt. Process until the mixture comes together.
3. Roll mixture into small balls and refrigerate for at least 1 hour until firm.
4. Serve chilled.

Nutritional Facts (Per Serving): Calories: 400 | Sugars: 22g | Fat: 24g | Carbohydrates: 38g | Protein: 10g | Fiber: 8g | Sodium: 30mg

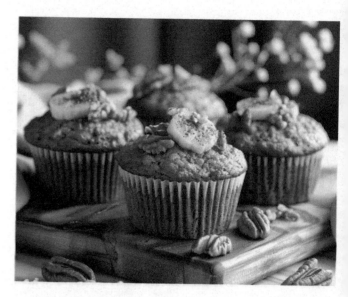

Banana and Walnut Muffins

Prep: 15 minutes | Cook: 25 minutes | Serves: 8

Ingredients:

- 2 cups whole wheat flour (240g)
- 1 tsp baking powder (5g)
- 1/2 tsp baking soda (2.5g)
- 1/2 tsp salt (2.5g)
- 1/2 cup walnuts, chopped (60g)
- 2 ripe bananas, mashed (240g)
- 1/2 cup almond butter (120g)
- 1/4 cup honey or low carb sweetener (60ml)
- 1/4 cup almond milk (60ml)
- 1 tsp vanilla extract (5ml)

Instructions:

1. Preheat oven to 350°F (175°C). Line a muffin tin with paper liners.
2. In a large bowl, mix whole wheat flour, baking powder, baking soda, salt, and chopped walnuts.
3. In another bowl, combine mashed bananas, almond butter, honey, almond milk, and vanilla extract.
4. Add wet ingredients to dry ingredients and mix until just combined.
5. Divide the batter evenly among the muffin cups.
6. Bake for 20-25 minutes until a toothpick inserted into the center comes out clean.

Nutritional Facts (Per Serving): Calories: 400 | Sugars: 15g | Fat: 20g | Carbohydrates: 50g | Protein: 8g | Fiber: 6g | Sodium: 200mg

CHAPTER 16: DINNER: Vibrant Salads and Bowls

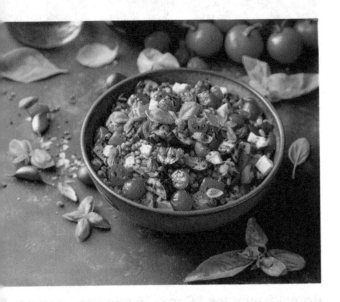

Farro Salad with Roasted Vegetables

Prep: 20 minutes | Cook: 30 minutes | Serves: 4

Ingredients:

- 1 cup farro (200g)
- 2 cups assorted vegetables (bell peppers, zucchini, cherry tomatoes) (400g)
- 2 tbsp olive oil (30ml)
- 1 tsp low carb sweetener
- Juice and zest of 1 lemon
- 1/4 cup crumbled feta cheese (40g)
- Salt and pepper to taste
- 1/4 cup chopped fresh parsley (15g)

Instructions:

1. Preheat oven to 400°F (200°C). Cook farro according to package instructions.
2. Toss vegetables with olive oil, salt, and pepper. Roast for 20-25 minutes until tender.
3. In a large bowl, combine cooked farro, roasted vegetables, lemon juice, zest, and low carb sweetener. Sprinkle with feta cheese and fresh parsley before serving.

Nutritional Facts (Per Serving): Calories: 400 | Carbs: 6g | Protein: 25g | Fat: 42g | Sodium: 4000mg

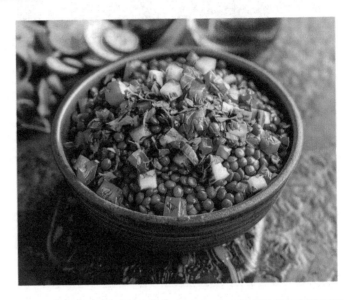

Lentil and Bulgur Wheat Salad

Prep: 20 minutes | Cook: 25 minutes | Serves: 4

Ingredients:

- 1/2 cup green lentils (100g)
- 1/2 cup bulgur wheat (100g)
- 2 cups vegetable broth (500ml)
- 1/2 cup diced cucumber (75g)
- 1/2 cup diced tomatoes (75g)
- 1/4 cup chopped red onion (40g)
- 2 tbsp olive oil (30ml)
- Juice of 1 lemon
- 1 tsp low carb sweetener
- 1/4 cup chopped fresh mint (15g)
- Salt and pepper to taste

Instructions:

1. Cook lentils in boiling water for 20-25 minutes until tender. Cook bulgur in vegetable broth for 10-12 minutes until soft.
2. In a large bowl, combine lentils, bulgur, cucumber, tomatoes, and red onion.
3. Whisk together olive oil, lemon juice, low carb sweetener, salt, and pepper. Pour over salad and mix well.

Nutritional Information (Per Serving): Calories: 400 | Sugars: 4g | Fat: 12g | Carbohydrates: 58g | Protein: 14g | Fiber: 12g | Sodium: 300mg

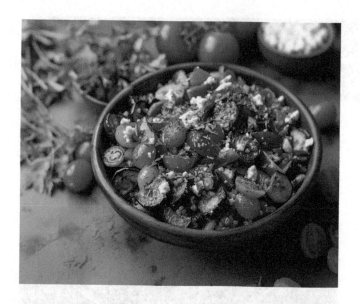

Roasted Vegetable and Millet Salad

Prep: 15 minutes | Cook: 30 minutes | Serves: 4

Ingredients:

- 1 cup millet (200g)
- 2 cups assorted vegetables (sweet potatoes, carrots, red onions) (400g)
- 2 tbsp olive oil (30ml)
- 1 tsp low carb sweetener
- Juice and zest of 1 orange
- 1/4 cup toasted pumpkin seeds (40g)
- Salt and pepper to taste
- 1/4 cup chopped fresh cilantro (15g)

Instructions:

1. Preheat oven to 400°F (200°C). Cook millet according to package instructions.
2. Toss vegetables with olive oil, salt, and pepper. Roast for 25-30 minutes until tender.
3. In a large bowl, combine cooked millet, roasted vegetables, orange juice, zest, and low carb sweetener.
4. Sprinkle with toasted pumpkin seeds and fresh cilantro before serving.

Nutritional Facts (Per Serving): Calories: 400 | Sugars: 7g | Fat: 14g | Carbohydrates: 57g | Protein: 10g | Fiber: 8g | Sodium: 350mg

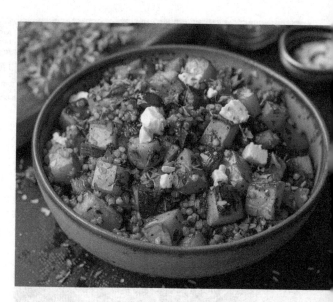

Freekeh and Roasted Root Vegetable Salad

Prep: 20 minutes | Cook: 30 minutes | Serves: 4

Ingredients:

- 1 cup freekeh (200g)
- 2 cups assorted root vegetables (carrots, parsnips, beets) (400g)
- 2 tbsp olive oil (30ml)
- 1 tsp low carb sweetener
- Juice and zest of 1 lemon
- 1/4 cup crumbled goat cheese (40g)
- Salt and pepper to taste
- 1/4 cup chopped fresh parsley (15g)

Instructions:

1. Preheat oven to 400°F (200°C). Cook freekeh according to package instructions.
2. Toss root vegetables with olive oil, salt, and pepper. Roast for 25-30 minutes until tender.
3. In a large bowl, combine cooked freekeh, roasted vegetables, lemon juice, zest, and low carb sweetener.
4. Sprinkle with goat cheese and fresh parsley before serving.

Nutritional Facts (Per Serving): Calories: 400 | Sugars: 7g | Fat: 14g | Carbohydrates: 56g | Protein: 11g | Fiber: 10g | Sodium: 350mg

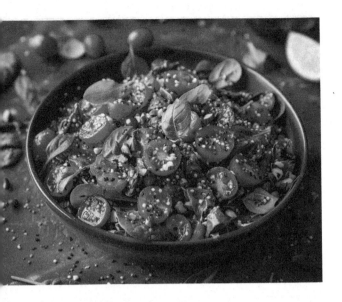

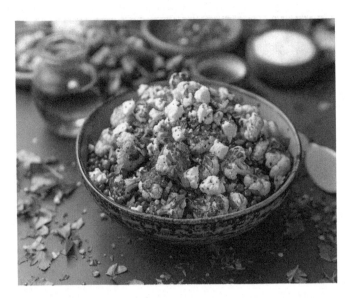

Amaranth and Spinach Salad

Prep: 15 minutes | Cook: 20 minutes | Serves: 4

Ingredients:

- 1 cup amaranth (200g)
- 4 cups fresh spinach (120g)
- 1/2 cup cherry tomatoes, halved (75g)
- 1/4 cup red onion, thinly sliced (40g)
- 2 tbsp olive oil (30ml)
- Juice of 1 lime
- 1 tsp low carb sweetener
- Salt and pepper to taste
- 1/4 cup chopped fresh basil (15g)

Instructions:

1. Cook amaranth in boiling water for 20 minutes until tender. Drain and let cool.
2. In a large bowl, combine cooked amaranth, spinach, cherry tomatoes, and red onion.
3. Whisk together olive oil, lime juice, low carb sweetener, salt, and pepper. Pour over salad and toss well.
4. Garnish with fresh basil before serving.

Nutritional Information (Per Serving): Calories: 400 | Sugars: 4g | Fat: 14g | Carbohydrates: 56g | Protein: 12g | Fiber: 8g | Sodium: 300mg

Roasted Cauliflower and Lentil Bowl

Prep: 15 minutes | Cook: 30 minutes | Serves: 4

Ingredients:

- 1 cup green or brown lentils (200g)
- 1 large head of cauliflower, chopped (600g)
- 2 tbsp olive oil (30ml)
- 1 tsp low carb sweetener
- 1 tsp ground cumin
- 1/2 tsp paprika
- Salt and pepper to taste
- 1/4 cup tahini sauce (60ml)
- Juice of 1 lemon
- 1/4 cup chopped fresh cilantro (15g)

Instructions:

1. Preheat oven to 425°F (220°C). Cook lentils in boiling water for 20-25 minutes until tender. Drain and set aside.
2. Toss cauliflower with olive oil, cumin, paprika, salt, and pepper. Roast for 25-30 minutes until golden brown.
3. In a large bowl, combine cooked lentils and roasted cauliflower. Drizzle with tahini sauce and lemon juice. Toss well.
4. Garnish with fresh cilantro before serving.

Nutritional Facts (Per Serving): Calories: 400 | Sugars: 5g | Fat: 14g | Carbohydrates: 50g | Protein: 16g | Fiber: 14g | Sodium: 300mg

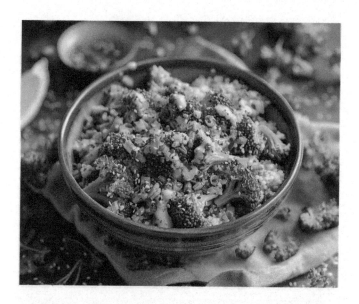

Millet and Broccoli Salad with Tahini Dressing

Prep: 15 minutes | Cook: 25 minutes | Serves: 4

Ingredients:

- 1 cup millet (200g)
- 2 cups broccoli florets (300g)
- 1/4 cup tahini (60g)
- 2 tbsp olive oil (30ml)
- Juice of 1 lemon
- 1 tsp low carb sweetener
- 1/4 cup chopped fresh parsley (15g)
- Salt and pepper to taste

Instructions:

1. Cook millet according to package instructions. Steam broccoli until tender, about 5-7 minutes.
2. In a small bowl, whisk together tahini, olive oil, lemon juice, low carb sweetener, salt, and pepper.
3. In a large bowl, combine cooked millet and broccoli. Drizzle with tahini dressing and toss to coat.
4. Garnish with fresh parsley before serving.

Nutritional Information (Per Serving): Calories: 400 | Sugars: 4g | Fat: 14g | Carbohydrates: 56g | Protein: 12g | Fiber: 9g | Sodium: 200mg

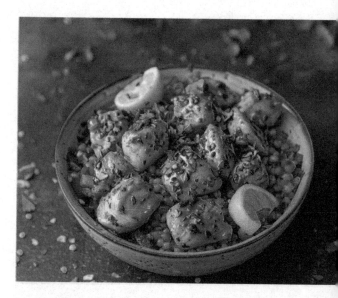

Lemon Garlic Chicken and Barley Salad

Prep: 15 minutes | Cook: 30 minutes | Serves: 4

Ingredients:

- 2 cups cooked barley (400g)
- 2 chicken breasts (300g each)
- 2 tbsp olive oil (30ml)
- Juice and zest of 1 lemon
- 2 garlic cloves, minced
- 1 cup cherry tomatoes, halved (150g)
- 1/4 cup chopped fresh basil (15g)
- Salt and pepper to taste

Instructions:

1. Cook barley according to package instructions. Season chicken breasts with salt, pepper, lemon zest, and garlic.
2. In a skillet, heat olive oil over medium heat. Cook chicken until golden and cooked through, about 6-7 minutes per side. Let rest and slice.
3. In a large bowl, combine cooked barley, cherry tomatoes, and sliced chicken. Drizzle with lemon juice and toss to coat.
4. Garnish with fresh basil before serving.

Nutritional Facts (Per Serving): Calories: 400 | Sugars: 3g | Fat: 14g | Carbohydrates: 38g | Protein: 30g | Fiber: 8g | Sodium: 250mg

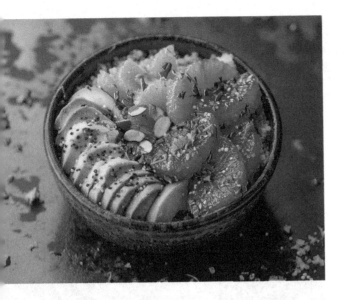

Citrus Avocado Quinoa Salad

Prep: 15 minutes | Cook: 20 minutes | Serves: 4

Ingredients:

- 1 cup quinoa (200g)
- 1 avocado, diced (150g)
- 1 orange, segmented
- 1 grapefruit, segmented
- 2 tbsp olive oil (30ml)
- Juice of 1 lime
- 1 tsp low carb sweetener
- 1/4 cup chopped fresh mint (15g)
- Salt and pepper to taste

Instructions:

1. Cook quinoa according to package instructions. Let cool.
2. In a large bowl, combine quinoa, avocado, orange, and grapefruit segments.
3. In a small bowl, whisk together olive oil, lime juice, low carb sweetener, salt, and pepper. Pour over salad and toss gently.
4. Garnish with fresh mint before serving.

Nutritional Information (Per Serving): Calories: 400 | Sugars: 6g | Fat: 18g | Carbohydrates: 50g | Protein: 8g | Fiber: 10g | Sodium: 150mg

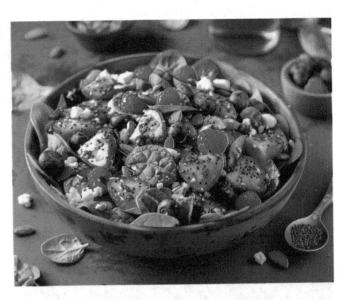

Mixed Berry and Baby Spinach Salad with Poppy Seed Dressing

Prep: 15 minutes | Serves: 4

Ingredients:

- 6 cups baby spinach (180g)
- 1 cup mixed berries (strawberries, blueberries, raspberries) (150g)
- 1/4 cup crumbled feta cheese (40g)
- 1/4 cup chopped pecans (30g)
- 2 tbsp poppy seeds (20g)
- 2 tbsp olive oil (30ml)
- 2 tbsp apple cider vinegar (30ml)
- 1 tsp low carb sweetener
- Salt and pepper to taste

Instructions:

1. In a large bowl, combine baby spinach, mixed berries, feta cheese, and pecans.
2. In a small bowl, whisk together poppy seeds, olive oil, apple cider vinegar, low carb sweetener, salt, and pepper.
3. Drizzle the dressing over the salad and toss gently to combine.

Nutritional Facts (Per Serving): Calories: 400 | Sugars: 8g | Fat: 28g | Carbohydrates: 26g | Protein: 6g | Fiber: 8g | Sodium: 200mg

CHAPTER 17: DINNER: Flavorful Seafood Dishes

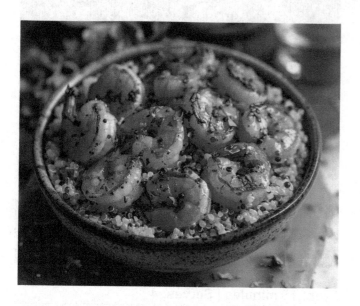

Lemon Garlic Shrimp and Quinoa

Prep: 15 minutes | Cook: 20 minutes | Serves: 4

Ingredients:

- 1 cup quinoa (200g)
- 1 lb large shrimp, peeled and deveined (450g)
- 2 tbsp olive oil (30ml)
- Juice and zest of 1 lemon
- 3 garlic cloves, minced
- 1/4 cup chopped fresh parsley (15g)
- Salt and pepper to taste

Instructions:

1. Cook quinoa according to package instructions.
2. In a large skillet, heat olive oil over medium heat. Add garlic and sauté for 1 minute.
3. Add shrimp, lemon juice, and zest, cooking until shrimp is pink and opaque, about 4-5 minutes.
4. In a large bowl, combine cooked quinoa, shrimp, and fresh parsley. Toss gently to combine. Season with salt and pepper to taste.

Nutritional Facts (Per Serving): Calories: 400 | Sugars: 2g | Fat: 14g | Carbohydrates: 32g | Protein: 32g | Fiber: 4g | Sodium: 500mg

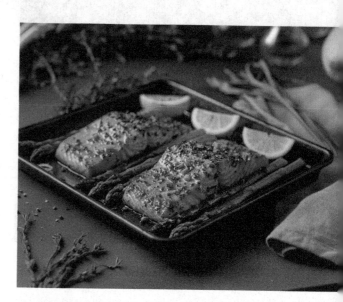

Herb-Crusted Salmon with Asparagus

Prep: 15 minutes | Cook: 20 minutes | Serves: 4

Ingredients:

- 4 salmon fillets (150g each)
- 2 tbsp olive oil (30ml)
- 1 tbsp chopped fresh dill (5g)
- 1 tbsp chopped fresh parsley (5g)
- 2 garlic cloves, minced
- Zest of 1 lemon
- 1 lb asparagus, trimmed (450g)
- Salt and pepper to taste

Instructions:

1. Preheat oven to 400°F (200°C). In a small bowl, mix olive oil, dill, parsley, garlic, and lemon zest.
2. Place salmon fillets on a baking sheet. Brush herb mixture over the salmon.
3. Arrange asparagus around salmon, drizzling with a little olive oil and seasoning with salt and pepper.
4. Bake for 15-20 minutes, until salmon is cooked through and asparagus is tender.

Nutritional Facts: Calories: 400 | Sugars: 1g | Fat: 24g | Carbohydrates: 8g | Protein: 34g | Fiber: 4g | Sodium: 300mg

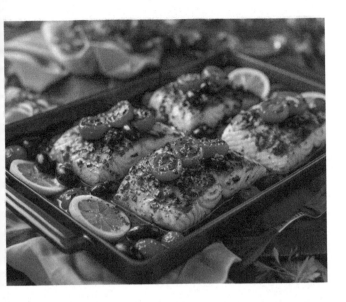

Mediterranean Baked Fish with Olives and Tomatoes

Prep: 15 minutes | Cook: 25 minutes | Serves: 4

Ingredients:

- 4 white fish fillets (150g each)
- 1 cup cherry tomatoes, halved (150g)
- 1/2 cup sliced olives (75g)
- 1/4 cup red onion, thinly sliced (40g)
- 2 tbsp olive oil (30ml)
- Juice of 1 lemon
- 1 tsp dried oregano
- Salt and pepper to taste

Instructions:

1. Preheat oven to 375°F (190°C).
2. Place fish fillets in a baking dish. Top with cherry tomatoes, olives, and red onion.
3. Drizzle with olive oil and lemon juice. Sprinkle with oregano, salt, and pepper.
4. Bake for 20-25 minutes, until fish is cooked through and flaky.

Nutritional Facts (Per Serving): Calories: 400 | Sugars: 2g | Fat: 20g | Carbohydrates: 6g | Protein: 44g | Fiber: 2g | Sodium: 600mg

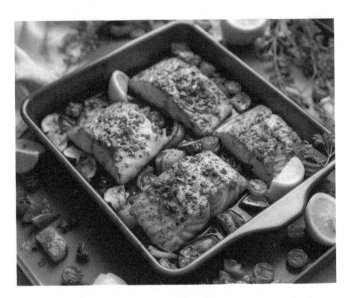

Turmeric Roasted Cod with Veggies

Prep: 15 minutes | Cook: 30 minutes | Serves: 4

Ingredients:

- 4 cod fillets (150g each)
- 2 cups broccoli florets (300g)
- 1 cup baby carrots (150g)
- 2 tbsp olive oil (30ml)
- 1 tsp ground turmeric
- 1/2 tsp ground cumin
- Juice of 1 lemon
- Salt and pepper to taste

Instructions:

1. Preheat oven to 400°F (200°C).
2. Toss broccoli and carrots with 1 tbsp olive oil, turmeric, cumin, salt, and pepper. Spread on a baking sheet.
3. Place cod fillets on top of vegetables. Drizzle with remaining olive oil and lemon juice.
4. Roast for 25-30 minutes, until fish is cooked through and vegetables are tender.

Nutritional Facts (Per Serving): Calories: 400 | Sugars: 5g | Fat: 14g | Carbohydrates: 24g | Protein: 44g | Fiber: 8g | Sodium: 400mg

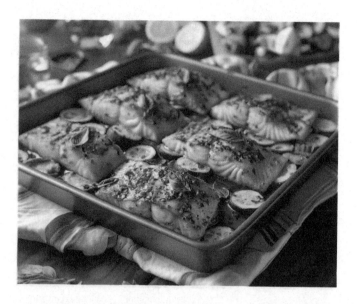

Lemon Basil Tilapia with Zucchini

Prep: 15 minutes | Cook: 20 minutes | Serves: 4

Ingredients:

- 4 tilapia fillets (150g each)
- 2 medium zucchinis, sliced (300g)
- 2 tbsp olive oil (30ml)
- Juice and zest of 1 lemon
- 2 tbsp chopped fresh basil (10g)
- Salt and pepper to taste

Instructions:

1. Preheat oven to 375°F (190°C).
2. Place tilapia fillets and zucchini slices in a baking dish. Drizzle with olive oil, lemon juice, and zest.
3. Season with salt and pepper. Sprinkle with fresh basil.
4. Bake for 15-20 minutes, until fish is cooked through and zucchini is tender.

Nutritional Facts (Per Serving): Calories: 400 | Sugars: 4g | Fat: 18g | Carbohydrates: 12g | Protein: 48g | Fiber: 4g | Sodium: 350mg

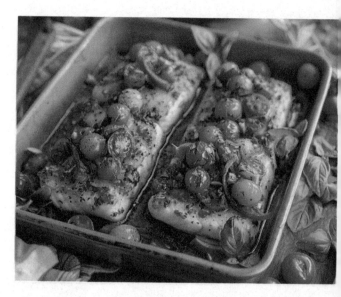

Baked Haddock with Tomato Relish

Prep: 15 minutes | Cook: 20 minutes | Serves: 4

Ingredients:

- 4 haddock fillets (150g each)
- 1 cup cherry tomatoes, halved (150g)
- 1/4 cup red onion, finely chopped (40g)
- 2 tbsp olive oil (30ml)
- Juice of 1 lemon
- 1 tsp low carb sweetener
- 1 tbsp chopped fresh basil (5g)
- Salt and pepper to taste

Instructions:

1. Preheat oven to 375°F (190°C).
2. Place haddock fillets in a baking dish. Drizzle with olive oil and lemon juice. Season with salt and pepper.
3. In a bowl, combine cherry tomatoes, red onion, low carb sweetener, and fresh basil. Spoon tomato relish over haddock fillets.
4. Bake for 20 minutes, until fish is cooked through and flakes easily with a fork.

Nutritional Facts (Per Serving): Calories: 400 | Sugars: 3g | Fat: 14g | Carbohydrates: 10g | Protein: 54g | Fiber: 2g | Sodium: 300mg

CHAPTER 18: DINNER: Comforting Casseroles and Bakes

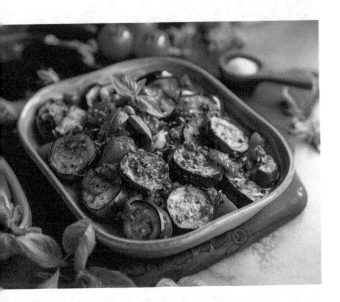

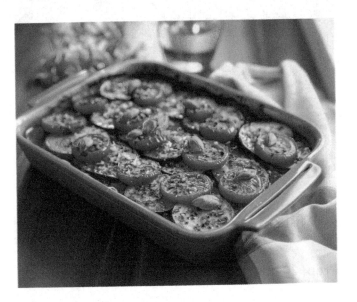

Mediterranean Eggplant Bake

Prep: 20 minutes | Cook: 40 minutes | Serves: 4

Ingredients:

- 2 medium eggplants, sliced (500g)
- 1 cup cherry tomatoes, halved (150g)
- 1/2 cup feta cheese, crumbled (75g)
- 1/4 cup olive oil (60ml)
- 2 garlic cloves, minced
- 1 tsp dried oregano
- Salt and pepper to taste
- 1/4 cup chopped fresh parsley (15g)

Instructions:

1. Preheat oven to 375°F (190°C).
2. Arrange eggplant slices in a baking dish. Drizzle with olive oil and sprinkle with minced garlic, oregano, salt, and pepper.
3. Top with cherry tomatoes and crumbled feta cheese.
4. Bake for 35-40 minutes, until eggplant is tender and cheese is golden. Garnish with fresh parsley before serving.

Nutritional Facts (Per Serving): Calories: 400 | Sugars: 7g | Fat: 28g | Carbohydrates: 25g | Protein: 10g | Fiber: 10g | Sodium: 400mg

Zucchini and Tomato Bake with Parmesan

Prep: 15 minutes | Cook: 30 minutes | Serves: 4

Ingredients:

- 3 medium zucchinis, sliced (450g)
- 1 cup cherry tomatoes, halved (150g)
- 1/2 cup grated Parmesan cheese (50g)
- 2 tbsp olive oil (30ml)
- 1 tsp dried basil
- Salt and pepper to taste
- 1/4 cup chopped fresh basil (15g)

Instructions:

1. Preheat oven to 375°F (190°C).
2. Arrange zucchini and cherry tomato slices in a baking dish. Drizzle with olive oil and sprinkle with dried basil, salt, and pepper.
3. Top with grated Parmesan cheese.
4. Bake for 25-30 minutes, until vegetables are tender and cheese is golden. Garnish with fresh basil before serving.

Nutritional Facts (Per Serving): Calories: 400 | Sugars: 6g | Fat: 28g | Carbohydrates: 18g | Protein: 14g | Fiber: 6g | Sodium: 500mg

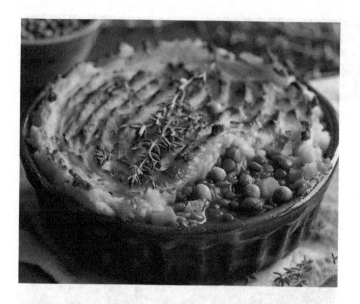

Lentil and Vegetable Shepherd's Pie

Prep: 20 minutes | Cook: 45 minutes | Serves: 4

Ingredients:

- 1 cup green lentils (200g)
- 2 cups vegetable broth (480ml)
- 1 cup diced carrots (150g)
- 1 cup diced celery (150g)
- 1 cup diced onion (150g)
- 2 cups mashed potatoes (400g)
- 2 tbsp olive oil (30ml)
- 1 tbsp tomato paste (15g)
- 1 tsp dried thyme
- Salt and pepper to taste

Instructions:

1. Preheat oven to 375°F (190°C). Cook lentils in vegetable broth until tender, about 20 minutes.
2. In a skillet, heat olive oil over medium heat. Sauté carrots, celery, and onion until soft, about 10 minutes. Stir in tomato paste, thyme, salt, and pepper.
3. Combine cooked lentils with sautéed vegetables and transfer to a baking dish. Spread mashed potatoes evenly on top.
4. Bake for 25 minutes, until the top is golden brown.

Nutritional Facts (Per Serving): Calories: 400 | Sugars: 7g | Fat: 10g | Carbohydrates: 65g | Protein: 12g | Fiber: 15g | Sodium: 400mg

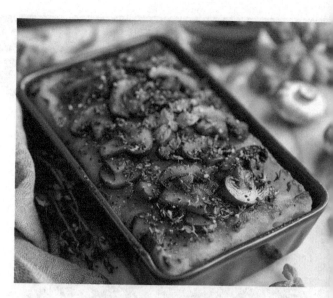

Baked Polenta with Marinara and Mushrooms

Prep: 15 minutes | Cook: 40 minutes | Serves: 4

Ingredients:

- 1 cup polenta (200g)
- 4 cups water (960ml)
- 1 cup marinara sauce (250g)
- 2 cups sliced mushrooms (300g)
- 1/4 cup grated Parmesan cheese (25g)
- 2 tbsp olive oil (30ml)
- 1 tsp dried oregano
- Salt and pepper to taste
- 1/4 cup chopped fresh basil (15g)

Instructions:

1. Preheat oven to 375°F (190°C). Cook polenta in boiling water until thickened, about 15 minutes. Spread in a baking dish and let cool.
2. In a skillet, heat olive oil over medium heat. Sauté mushrooms until soft, about 10 minutes. Season with oregano, salt, and pepper.
3. Spread marinara sauce over polenta, top with sautéed mushrooms, and sprinkle with Parmesan cheese.
4. Bake for 25 minutes, until golden and bubbly. Garnish with fresh basil before serving.

Nutritional Facts (Per Serving): Calories: 400 | Sugars: 6g | Fat: 14g | Carbohydrates: 60g | Protein: 10g | Fiber: 7g | Sodium: 600mg

CHAPTER 19: DINNER: Family-Style Dinner Ideas

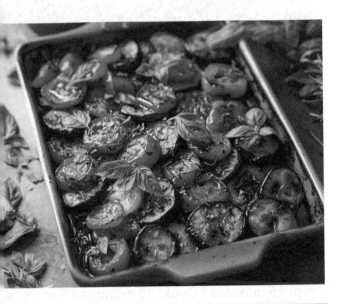

Ratatouille with Fresh Herbs

Prep: 20 minutes | Cook: 40 minutes | Serves: 4

Ingredients:

- 1 eggplant, diced (300g)
- 1 zucchini, diced (200g)
- 1 red bell pepper, diced (150g)
- 1 yellow bell pepper, diced (150g)
- 1 cup cherry tomatoes, halved (150g)
- 1 onion, diced (150g)
- 3 garlic cloves, minced
- 2 tbsp olive oil (30ml)
- 1 tsp dried thyme
- 1 tsp dried oregano
- Salt and pepper to taste
- 1/4 cup chopped fresh parsley (15g)

Instructions:

1. Preheat oven to 375°F (190°C). In a large bowl, toss eggplant, zucchini, bell peppers, cherry tomatoes, and onion with olive oil, garlic, thyme, oregano, salt, and pepper.
2. Spread the vegetable mixture in a baking dish.
3. Bake for 40 minutes, stirring halfway through, until vegetables are tender and slightly caramelized.
4. Garnish with fresh parsley before serving.

Nutritional Facts (Per Serving): Calories: 400 | Sugars: 10g | Fat: 18g | Carbohydrates: 50g | Protein: 6g | Fiber: 12g | Sodium: 350mg

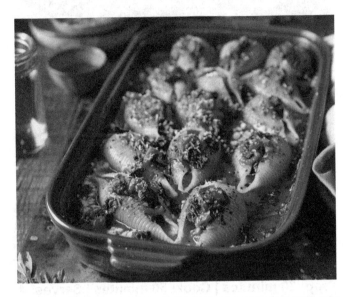

Spinach and Ricotta Stuffed Shells

Prep: 20 minutes | Cook: 30 minutes | Serves: 4

Ingredients:

- 12 jumbo pasta shells (120g)
- 2 cups ricotta cheese (450g)
- 2 cups fresh spinach, chopped (60g)
- 1 egg (50g)
- 2 cups marinara sauce (500ml)
- 1/4 cup grated Parmesan cheese (25g)
- 1 tbsp olive oil (15ml)
- Salt and pepper to taste

Instructions:

1. Preheat oven to 375°F (190°C). Cook pasta shells according to package instructions.
2. In a bowl, mix ricotta, spinach, egg, salt, and pepper. Stuff each shell with the mixture.
3. Spread 1 cup marinara sauce in a baking dish. Arrange stuffed shells on top, cover with remaining sauce, and sprinkle with Parmesan.
4. Drizzle with olive oil and bake for 25-30 minutes, until bubbly and golden.

Nutritional Facts (Per Serving): Calories: 400 | Sugars: 6g | Fat: 20g | Carbohydrates: 30g | Protein: 20g | Fiber: 4g | Sodium: 600mg

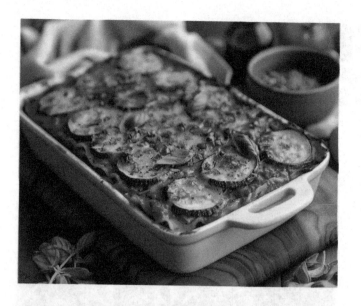

Vegan Lasagna with Cashew Cheese

Prep: 30 minutes | Cook: 50 minutes | Serves: 4

Ingredients:

- 9 lasagna noodles (200g)
- 3 cups marinara sauce (750ml)
- 1 cup cashews, soaked (150g)
- 1/4 cup nutritional yeast (20g)
- 1 tbsp lemon juice (15ml)
- 1 garlic clove
- 2 cups spinach, chopped (60g)
- 1 zucchini, sliced (200g)
- 1 bell pepper, diced (150g)
- Salt and pepper to taste

Instructions:

1. Preheat oven to 375°F (190°C). Cook lasagna noodles according to package instructions.
2. In a blender, combine cashews, nutritional yeast, lemon juice, garlic, salt, and 1/2 cup water to make cashew cheese.
3. Spread a layer of marinara sauce in a baking dish. Layer noodles, cashew cheese, spinach, zucchini, and bell pepper. Repeat layers, ending with marinara sauce.
4. Bake for 45-50 minutes, until vegetables are tender and sauce is bubbly.

Nutritional Facts (Per Serving): Calories: 400 | Sugars: 8g | Fat: 18g | Carbohydrates: 50g | Protein: 12g | Fiber: 8g | Sodium: 500mg

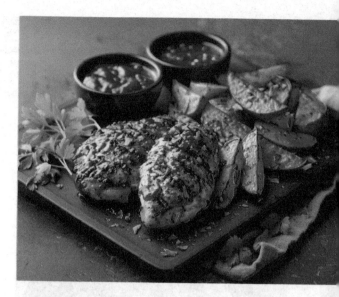

BBQ Chicken and Sweet Potato Wedges

Prep: 15 minutes | Cook: 30 minutes | Serves: 4

Ingredients:

- 2 boneless, skinless chicken breasts (300g each)
- 1/2 cup BBQ sauce (120ml)
- 2 large sweet potatoes, cut into wedges (600g)
- 2 tbsp olive oil (30ml)
- 1 tsp paprika
- 1/2 tsp garlic powder
- Salt and pepper to taste

Instructions:

1. Preheat oven to 400°F (200°C). Toss sweet potato wedges with olive oil, paprika, garlic powder, salt, and pepper. Spread on a baking sheet and bake for 25-30 minutes, until tender.
2. Brush chicken breasts with BBQ sauce and bake on a separate baking sheet for 20-25 minutes, until cooked through.
3. Serve chicken with sweet potato wedges.

Nutritional Facts (Per Serving): Calories: 400 | Sugars: 12g | Fat: 12g | Carbohydrates: 40g | Protein: 30g | Fiber: 6g | Sodium: 700mg

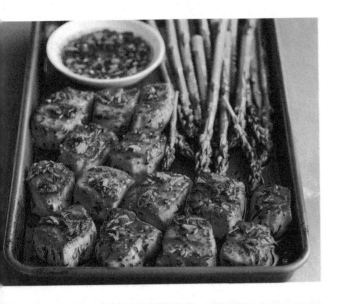

Herb Marinated Pork Tenderloin with Asparagus

Prep: 15 minutes | Cook: 25 minutes | Serves: 4

Ingredients:

- 1.5 lbs pork tenderloin (680g)
- 2 tbsp olive oil (30ml)
- 2 tbsp chopped fresh rosemary (10g)
- 2 tbsp chopped fresh thyme (10g)
- 3 garlic cloves, minced
- Juice of 1 lemon
- 1 lb asparagus, trimmed (450g)
- Salt and pepper to taste

Instructions:

1. Preheat oven to 400°F (200°C).
2. Marinate pork tenderloin with olive oil, rosemary, thyme, garlic, lemon juice, salt, and pepper for 10 minutes.
3. Place tenderloin in a baking dish and roast for 20-25 minutes, until the internal temperature reaches 145°F (63°C).
4. During the last 10 minutes of roasting, add asparagus to the baking dish, tossing with a little olive oil, salt, and pepper.
5. Let the pork rest for 5 minutes before slicing and serving with asparagus.

Nutritional Facts (Per Serving): Calories: 400 | Sugars: 2g | Fat: 18g | Carbohydrates: 10g | Protein: 48g | Fiber: 4g | Sodium: 300mg

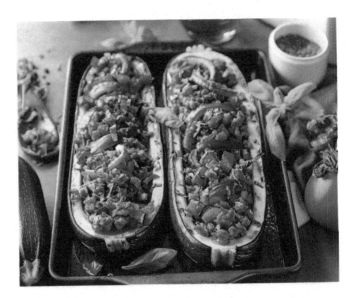

Ground Turkey and Veggie Stuffed Zucchini

Prep: 15 minutes | Cook: 30 minutes | Serves: 4

Ingredients:

- 4 medium zucchinis (800g)
- 1 lb ground turkey (450g)
- 1 cup diced bell peppers (150g)
- 1 cup diced tomatoes (150g)
- 1/2 cup diced onion (75g)
- 2 tbsp olive oil (30ml)
- 1 tsp dried oregano
- 1 tsp dried basil
- 1/2 cup shredded mozzarella cheese (50g)
- Salt and pepper to taste

Instructions:

1. Preheat oven to 375°F (190°C). Slice zucchinis in half lengthwise and scoop out the centers to create boats.
2. In a skillet, heat olive oil over medium heat. Sauté onion, bell peppers, and tomatoes until soft, about 5 minutes. Add ground turkey, oregano, basil, salt, and pepper, cooking until turkey is browned, about 7 minutes.
3. Stuff zucchini boats with the turkey and veggie mixture. Place in a baking dish and sprinkle with mozzarella cheese.
4. Bake for 20-25 minutes, until zucchini is tender and cheese is melted and golden.

Nutritional Facts (Per Serving): Calories: 400 | Sugars: 7g | Fat: 22g | Carbohydrates: 20g | Protein: 35g | Fiber: 6g | Sodium: 400mg

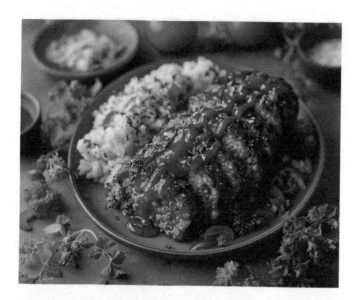

BBQ Turkey Meatloaf with Cauliflower Rice

Prep: 15 minutes | Cook: 45 minutes | Serves: 4

Ingredients:

- 1 lb ground turkey (450g)
- 1/2 cup BBQ sauce (120ml)
- 1/2 cup finely chopped onion (75g)
- 1/2 cup finely chopped bell pepper (75g)
- 1/4 cup breadcrumbs (30g)
- 1 egg (50g)
- 1 tsp garlic powder
- 1 tsp paprika
- Salt and pepper to taste
- 4 cups cauliflower rice (400g)

Instructions:

1. Preheat oven to 375°F (190°C). In a bowl, mix ground turkey, 1/4 cup BBQ sauce, onion, bell pepper, breadcrumbs, egg, garlic powder, paprika, salt, and pepper.
2. Shape mixture into a loaf and place in a baking dish. Brush the top with the remaining BBQ sauce.
3. Bake for 40-45 minutes, until internal temperature reaches 165°F (74°C).
4. Meanwhile, cook cauliflower rice in a skillet over medium heat until tender, about 5-7 minutes. Season with salt and pepper.
5. Serve sliced meatloaf with cauliflower rice.

Nutritional Facts (Per Serving): Calories: 400 | Sugars: 8g | Fat: 15g | Carbohydrates: 30g | Protein: 35g | Fiber: 6g | Sodium: 600mg

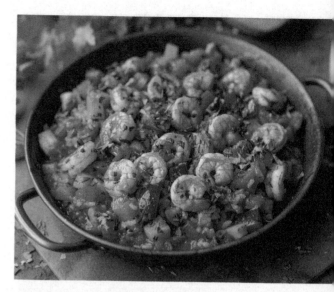

Anti-Inflammatory Paella

Prep: 20 minutes | Cook: 40 minutes | Serves: 4

Ingredients:

- 1 cup brown rice (200g)
- 1 lb chicken breast, diced (450g)
- 1/2 lb shrimp, peeled and deveined (225g)
- 1 red bell pepper, diced (150g)
- 1 yellow bell pepper, diced (150g)
- 1 cup green beans, chopped (150g)
- 1 cup diced tomatoes (150g)
- 4 cups chicken broth (960ml)
- 2 tbsp olive oil (30ml)
- 1 tsp turmeric
- 1 tsp smoked paprika
- 1/2 tsp saffron threads
- 3 garlic cloves, minced
- Salt and pepper to taste
- 1/4 cup chopped fresh parsley (15g)

Instructions:

1. Heat olive oil in a large skillet or paella pan over medium heat. Add chicken, cooking until browned, about 5-7 minutes. Remove and set aside.
2. In the same pan, sauté garlic, bell peppers, and green beans for 3-4 minutes. Stir in turmeric, smoked paprika, and saffron.
3. Add brown rice and diced tomatoes, stirring to coat. Pour in chicken broth and bring to a boil.
4. Return chicken to the pan and simmer for 20 minutes. Add shrimp and cook for an additional 10 minutes, until rice is tender and shrimp is cooked through. Season with salt and pepper.

Nutritional Facts (Per Serving): Calories: 400 | Sugars: 6g | Fat: 14g | Carbohydrates: 35g | Protein: 30g | Fiber: 5g | Sodium: 700mg

CHAPTER 20: BONUSES

Meal Plans and Shopping Templates

To elevate your anti-inflammatory diet journey, we've created a comprehensive 30-day grocery shopping guide, perfectly aligned with our cookbook. This guide simplifies meal preparation, emphasizing fresh, natural ingredients while minimizing processed foods. Be vigilant about hidden sugars, particularly in sauces and dressings. Adjust quantities according to your needs, embracing the anti-inflammatory focus on whole, nutrient-dense foods. Enjoy the path to healthy, delicious cooking!

Grocery Shopping List for 7-Day Meal Plan

Proteins

Eggs: 2 dozen (for Greek Yogurt and Feta Omelette, Curried Cauliflower and Egg Skillet, Zucchini and Bell Pepper Egg Muffins)
Greek Yogurt: 2 cups (for Greek Yogurt and Feta Omelette, Spinach and Ricotta Stuffed Crêpes)
Feta Cheese: 1 cup (for Greek Yogurt and Feta Omelette)
Shrimp: 1 pound (for Lemon Garlic Shrimp and Quinoa)
Chicken Breast: 2 (for Lemon Garlic Chicken and Barley Salad)
Salmon: 2 fillets (for Herb-Crusted Salmon with Asparagus)
Turkey: 1 pound (for BBQ Turkey Meatloaf with Cauliflower Rice)
Cod: 2 fillets (for Turmeric Roasted Cod with Veggies)

Dairy and Dairy Alternatives:

Greek Yogurt: 1 cup (for Mango and Turmeric Lassi, Cucumber and Dill Greek Yogurt Dip)
Coconut Milk: 1 can (for Coconut and Matcha Energy Bars)
Almond Milk: 1 quart (for Blueberry and Turmeric Oatmeal)

Fruits:

Avocado: 3 (for Avocado and Black Bean Stuffed Mini Peppers, Avocado and Cilantro Salsa)
Mango: 2 (for Mango and Turmeric Lassi, Avocado and Black Bean Stuffed Mini Peppers)
Blueberries: 1 pint (for Blueberry and Turmeric Oatmeal)
Pineapple: 1 (for Green Detox Smoothie with Kale and Pineapple)
Dates: 1 cup (for Almond Butter and Date Bars)
Lemons: 4 (for Lemon Garlic Shrimp and Quinoa, Lemon Garlic Chicken and Barley

Salad, Beet and Walnut Hummus with Crudités)

Vegetables & Herbs:

Spinach: 1 bunch (for Greek Yogurt and Feta Omelette, Spinach and Ricotta Stuffed Crêpes, Lentil and Bulgur Wheat Salad)
Carrots: 6 (for Creamy Carrot and Ginger Soup, Spicy Chickpea and Brown Rice Bowl)
Ginger: 1 knob (for Creamy Carrot and Ginger Soup, Mango and Turmeric Lassi)
Bell Peppers: 4 (for Zucchini and Bell Pepper Egg Muffins, Avocado and Black Bean Stuffed Mini Peppers)
Zucchini: 4 (for Zucchini and Bell Pepper Egg Muffins, Baked Polenta with Marinara and Mushrooms)
Cauliflower: 1 head (for Curried Cauliflower and Egg Skillet, Baked Falafel Balls)
Tomatoes: 6 (for Tomato Basil and Quinoa Soup, One-Pot Mediterranean Pasta with Olives)

Cucumbers: 2 (for Cucumber and Dill Greek Yogurt Dip)
Garlic: 2 bulbs (for various recipes)
Onions: 4 (for various recipes)
Kale: 1 bunch (for Green Detox Smoothie with Kale and Pineapple)
Eggplant: 2 (for Mediterranean Eggplant Bake)
Herbs: Fresh parsley, basil, cilantro (for various recipes)

Grains & Bakery:

Quinoa: 2 cups (for Lemon Garlic Shrimp and Quinoa, Quinoa and Black Bean Stuffed Peppers)
Brown Rice: 1 cup (for Spicy Chickpea and Brown Rice Bowl)
Barley: 1 cup (for Lemon Garlic Chicken and Barley Salad)
Whole Grain Bread: 1 loaf (for various recipes)
Polenta: 1 tube (for Baked Polenta with Marinara and Mushrooms)

Nuts & Seeds:

Almonds: 1 cup (for Almond Butter and Date Bars, Beet and Walnut Hummus with Crudités)
Walnuts: 1 cup (for Beet and Walnut Hummus with Crudités)
Chia Seeds: 1/2 cup (for various recipes)
Pumpkin Seeds: 1/2 cup (for Coconut and Matcha Energy Bars)

Pantry Staples:

Olive Oil: 1 bottle (for various recipes)

Coconut Oil: 1 jar (for Coconut and Matcha Energy Bars)
Low Carb Sweetener: 1 package (for various recipes)
Soy Sauce: 1 bottle (for One-Pot Mediterranean Pasta with Olives)
Balsamic Vinegar: 1 bottle (for Balsamic Glazed Chicken)
Paprika: 1 jar (for Classic Hummus with Paprika)
Turmeric: 1 jar (for Blueberry and Turmeric Oatmeal, Mango and Turmeric Lassi, Turmeric Roasted Cod with Veggies)
Ground Cinnamon: 1 jar (for various recipes)
Salt and Pepper: 1 set (for various recipes)

Miscellaneous:

Cocoa Powder: 1 container (for Coconut and Matcha Energy Bars)
Dark Chocolate: 1 bar (for Coconut and Matcha Energy Bars)
Vanilla Extract: 1 bottle (for various recipes)

> ## Grocery Shopping List for 8-14 Day Meal Plan

Proteins

Eggs: 2 dozen (for Asparagus and Goat Cheese Egg Bake, Avocado and Spinach Egg Scramble, Veggie and Cheese Breakfast Quesadilla, Mushroom and Swiss Chard Quiche)

Goat Cheese: 1 cup (for Asparagus and Goat Cheese Egg Bake)
Cottage Cheese: 1 cup (for Cottage Cheese and Berry Parfait)
Ground Turkey: 1 pound (for Ground Turkey and Veggie Stuffed Zucchini)
Chicken Breast: 2 (for Herb-Roasted Chicken with Quinoa Pilaf, Lemon Herb Chicken and Quinoa Salad)
Tilapia: 2 fillets (for Lemon Basi Tilapia with Zucchini)

Dairy and Dairy Alternatives:

Greek Yogurt: 1 cup (for various recipes)
Almond Milk: 1 quart (for Black Rice and Mango Porridge, Chia Seed Pudding with Almonds and Blueberries)
Cashew Cheese: 1 cup (for Vegan Lasagna with Cashew Cheese)
Cheddar Cheese: 1 cup (for One-Pot Broccoli and Cheddar Quinoa)
Butter: 1 stick (for various recipes)

Fruits:

Avocado: 3 (for Avocado and Spinach Egg Scramble, Artichoke and Spinach Yogurt Dip)
Berries: 1 pint (for Cottage Cheese and Berry Parfait, Chia Seed Pudding with Almonds and Blueberries)
Mango: 2 (for Black Rice and Mango Porridge)
Lemons: 4 (for Lemon Basil Tilapia with Zucchini, Lemon

Herb Chicken and Quinoa Salad, Artichoke and Spinach Yogurt Dip)
Bananas: 2 (for Pumpkin Spice and Flaxseed Oatmeal)
Dates: 1 cup (for Ginger and Turmeric Bliss Balls)

Vegetables & Herbs:

Asparagus: 1 bunch (for Asparagus and Goat Cheese Egg Bake)
Spinach: 2 bunches (for Avocado and Spinach Egg Scramble, Quinoa and Spinach Stuffed Tomatoes, Lentil and Vegetable Shepherd's Pie)
Zucchini: 6 (for Zucchini and Quinoa Bites, Ground Turkey and Veggie Stuffed Zucchini, Lemon Basil Tilapia with Zucchini)
Tomatoes: 6 (for Quinoa and Spinach Stuffed Tomatoes, Wild Rice and Cranberry Pilaf)
Green Beans: 1 pound (for One-Pot Green Bean and Potato Stew)
Potatoes: 4 (for One-Pot Green Bean and Potato Stew, Cauliflower Hash Browns with Poached Eggs)
Cauliflower: 1 head (for Cauliflower Hash Browns with Poached Eggs)
Pumpkin: 1 small (for Pumpkin and Chickpea Soup with Turmeric, Pumpkin Spice and Flaxseed Oatmeal)
Chickpeas: 3 cups (for Pumpkin and Chickpea Soup with Turmeric, Couscous and Chickpea Pilaf)
Swiss Chard: 1 bunch (for Mushroom and Swiss Chard Quiche)

Mushrooms: 1 pound (for Mushroom and Swiss Chard Quiche, One-Pot Vegetable and Barley Casserole)
Bell Peppers: 4 (for Veggie and Cheese Breakfast Quesadilla)
Cucumbers: 2 (for Cucumber and Dill Greek Yogurt Dip)
Eggplant: 2 (for Smoky Eggplant Baba Ganoush)
Herbs: Fresh parsley, basil, cilantro, dill (for various recipes)
Garlic: 2 bulbs (for various recipes)
Onions: 6 (for various recipes)
Kale: 1 bunch (for Green Detox Smoothie with Kale and Pineapple)
Root Vegetables: Carrots, beets, parsnips (for Freekeh and Roasted Root Vegetable Salad)
Artichokes: 1 can (for Artichoke and Spinach Yogurt Dip)

Grains & Bakery:

Quinoa: 2 cups (for Herb-Roasted Chicken with Quinoa Pilaf, Lemon Herb Chicken and Quinoa Salad)
Freekeh: 1 cup (for Freekeh and Roasted Root Vegetable Salad)
Barley: 1 cup (for One-Pot Vegetable and Barley Casserole)
Couscous: 1 cup (for Couscous and Chickpea Pilaf)
Wild Rice: 1 cup (for Wild Rice and Cranberry Pilaf)
Brown Rice: 1 cup (for Spicy Chickpea and Brown Rice Bowl)
Polenta: 1 tube (for Baked Polenta with Marinara and Mushrooms)

Black Rice: 1 cup (for Black Rice and Mango Porridge)
Whole Grain Bread: 1 loaf (for various recipes)

Nuts & Seeds:

Almonds: 1 cup (for Chia Seed Pudding with Almonds and Blueberries, Ginger and Turmeric Bliss Balls)
Walnuts: 1 cup (for Ginger and Turmeric Bliss Balls)
Chia Seeds: 1/2 cup (for Chia Seed Pudding with Almonds and Blueberries)
Pumpkin Seeds: 1/2 cup (for Ginger and Turmeric Bliss Balls)

Pantry Staples:

Olive Oil: 1 bottle (for various recipes)
Coconut Oil: 1 jar (for various recipes)
Low Carb Sweetener: 1 package (for various recipes)
Soy Sauce: 1 bottle (for One-Pot Mediterranean Pasta with Olives)
Balsamic Vinegar: 1 bottle (for Balsamic Glazed Chicken)
Paprika: 1 jar (for various recipes)
Turmeric: 1 jar (for Pumpkin Spice and Flaxseed Oatmeal, Ginger and Turmeric Bliss Balls)
Ground Cinnamon: 1 jar (for various recipes)
Salt and Pepper: 1 set (for various recipes)

Miscellaneous:

Cocoa Powder: 1 container (for Coconut and Matcha Energy Bars)

Dark Chocolate: 1 bar (for Ginger and Turmeric Bliss Balls)

Vanilla Extract: 1 bottle (for various recipes)

Grocery Shopping List for 15-21 Day Meal Plan

Proteins:

Chicken Breast: 3 (for Balsamic Chicken and Roasted Vegetables, BBQ Chicken and Sweet Potato Wedges)

Ground Turkey: 1 pound (for Spicy Turkey and Sweet Potato Skillet, Moroccan Spiced Turkey Meatballs)

Turkey Sausage: 1 pound (for Egg and Turkey Sausage Breakfast Muffins)

Haddock: 2 fillets (for Baked Haddock with Tomato Relish)

Pork Tenderloin: 1 pound (for Herb Marinated Pork Tenderloin with Asparagus)

Haddock: 2 fillets (for Mediterranean Baked Fish with Olives and Tomatoes)

Eggs: 2 dozen (for Turmeric Spiced Shakshuka, Egg and Turkey Sausage Breakfast Muffins)

Greek Yogurt: 2 cups (for Greek Yogurt Pancakes with Fresh Berries)

Dairy and Dairy Alternatives:

Greek Yogurt: 1 cup (for various recipes)

Almond Milk: 1 quart (for Berry and Beetroot Smoothie, Banana and Almond Porridge)

Feta Cheese: 1 cup (for Spinach and Ricotta Stuffed Shells)

Cheddar Cheese: 1 cup (for Sweet Potato and Kale Quesadillas)

Butter: 1 stick (for various recipes)

Fruits:

Berries: 1 pint (for Berry and Beetroot Smoothie, Greek Yogurt Pancakes with Fresh Berries)

Bananas: 2 (for Banana and Almond Porridge)

Kiwi: 2 (for Spinach and Kiwi Green Juice)

Apples: 3 (for Apple and Date Overnight Oats)

Dates: 1 cup (for Apple and Date Overnight Oats)

Avocado: 4 (for Mini Avocado Toasts with Tomato, Avocado and Cilantro Salsa)

Lemons: 4 (for Cashew and Herb Pesto, Baked Haddock with Tomato Relish, Apple and Date Overnight Oats)

Tomatoes: 6 (for Mini Avocado Toasts with Tomato, Roasted Red Pepper and Chickpea Crostini)

Vegetables & Herbs:

Spinach: 2 bunches (for One-Pot Creamy Tomato and Spinach Pasta, Spinach and Ricotta Stuffed Shells)

Sweet Potatoes: 4 (for Spicy Turkey and Sweet Potato Skillet, Sweet Potato and Kale Quesadillas)

Carrots: 6 (for Carrot and Cumin Fritters, Minestrone with Cannellini Beans and Kale)

Bell Peppers: 4 (for Quinoa and Black Bean Stuffed Peppers, Roasted Red Pepper and Chickpea Crostini)

Zucchini: 4 (for Balsamic Chicken and Roasted Vegetables, Lemon Basil Tilapia with Zucchini)

Kale: 1 bunch (for Sweet Potato and Kale Quesadillas)

Green Beans: 1 pound (for One-Pot Green Bean and Potato Stew)

Cauliflower: 1 head (for Cauliflower Hash Browns with Poached Eggs)

Garlic: 2 bulbs (for various recipes)

Onions: 6 (for various recipes)

Beets: 2 (for Berry and Beetroot Smoothie, Freekeh and Roasted Root Vegetable Salad)

Cilantro: 1 bunch (for Avocado and Cilantro Salsa)

Asparagus: 1 bunch (for Herb Marinated Pork Tenderloin with Asparagus)

Herbs: Fresh parsley, basil, dill (for various recipes)

Grains & Bakery:

Quinoa: 2 cups (for One-Pot Creamy Tomato and Spinach Pasta, Herb-Roasted Chicken with Quinoa Pilaf)

Barley: 1 cup (for One-Pot Vegetable and Barley Casserole)

Freekeh: 1 cup (for Freekeh and Roasted Root Vegetable Salad)
Couscous: 1 cup (for Couscous and Chickpea Pilaf)
Wild Rice: 1 cup (for Wild Rice and Cranberry Pilaf)
Brown Rice: 1 cup (for Spicy Chickpea and Brown Rice Bowl)
Polenta: 1 tube (for Baked Polenta with Marinara and Mushrooms)
Black Rice: 1 cup (for Black Rice and Mango Porridge)
Whole Grain Bread: 1 loaf (for Mini Avocado Toasts with Tomato)

Nuts & Seeds:

Almonds: 1 cup (for Banana and Almond Porridge, Ginger and Turmeric Bliss Balls)
Walnuts: 1 cup (for Ginger and Turmeric Bliss Balls)
Cashews: 1 cup (for Cashew and Herb Pesto)
Pumpkin Seeds: 1/2 cup (for Ginger and Turmeric Bliss Balls)

Pantry Staples:

Olive Oil: 1 bottle (for various recipes)
Coconut Oil: 1 jar (for various recipes)
Low Carb Sweetener: 1 package (for various recipes)
Soy Sauce: 1 bottle (for One-Pot Mediterranean Pasta with Olives)
Balsamic Vinegar: 1 bottle (for Balsamic Glazed Chicken)
Paprika: 1 jar (for various recipes)

Turmeric: 1 jar (for Pumpkin Spice and Flaxseed Oatmeal, Ginger and Turmeric Bliss Balls)
Ground Cinnamon: 1 jar (for various recipes)
Salt and Pepper: 1 set (for various recipes)

Miscellaneous:

Cocoa Powder: 1 container (for Coconut and Matcha Energy Bars)
Dark Chocolate: 1 bar (for Ginger and Turmeric Bliss Balls)
Vanilla Extract: 1 bottle (for various recipes)

Grocery Shopping List for 22-28 Day Meal Plan

Proteins:

Chicken Breast: 3 (for Balsamic Chicken and Roasted Vegetables, BBQ Turkey Meatloaf with Cauliflower Rice)
Ground Turkey: 1 pound (for Moroccan Spiced Turkey Meatballs, BBQ Turkey Meatloaf with Cauliflower Rice)
Turkey Sausage: 1 pound (for Egg and Turkey Sausage Breakfast Muffins)
Salmon: 2 fillets (for Herb-Crusted Salmon with Asparagus)
Tilapia: 2 fillets (for Lemon Basil Tilapia with Zucchini)
Cottage Cheese: 1 cup (for Almond Flour Waffles with Cottage Cheese)

Eggs: 2 dozen (for Broccoli and Cheddar Breakfast Casserole, Spinach and Mushroom Keto Quiche, Sweet Potato and Kale Quesadillas)

Dairy and Dairy Alternatives:

Cheddar Cheese: 1 cup (for Broccoli and Cheddar Breakfast Casserole)
Almond Milk: 1 quart (for Mixed Berry and Almond Smoothie, Cranberry and Pecan Porridge)
Greek Yogurt: 1 cup (for Cucumber and Dill Greek Yogurt Dip)
Butter: 1 stick (for various recipes)
Cashew Cheese: 1 cup (for Vegan Lasagna with Cashew Cheese)

Fruits:

Mixed Berries: 1 pint (for Mixed Berry and Almond Smoothie)
Lemons: 4 (for Lemon Poppy Seed Porridge, Beet and Walnut Hummus with Crudités, Lemon Basil Tilapia with Zucchini)
Avocado: 3 (for Mini Avocado Toasts with Tomato)
Cranberries: 1 cup (for Cranberry and Pecan Porridge)
Bananas: 2 (for Mixed Berry and Almond Smoothie)
Dates: 1 cup (for Ginger and Turmeric Bliss Balls)
Pecans: 1 cup (for Cranberry and Pecan Porridge)
Almonds: 1 cup (for Mixed Berry and Almond Smoothie, Ginger and Turmeric Bliss Balls)

Vegetables & Herbs:

Sweet Potatoes: 4 (for Sweet Potato and Kale Quesadillas)
Kale: 2 bunches (for Sweet Potato and Kale Quesadillas, Lentil and Bulgur Wheat Salad)
Broccoli: 1 head (for Broccoli and Cheddar Breakfast Casserole)
Spinach: 2 bunches (for Quinoa and Spinach Stuffed Tomatoes, Spinach and Mushroom Keto Quiche)
Tomatoes: 6 (for Mini Avocado Toasts with Tomato, Quinoa and Spinach Stuffed Tomatoes)
Carrots: 6 (for Carrot and Cumin Fritters, One-Pot Eggplant and Chickpea Tagine)
Bell Peppers: 4 (for Quinoa and Spinach Stuffed Tomatoes, One-Pot Mediterranean Pasta with Olives)
Zucchini: 4 (for Lemon Basil Tilapia with Zucchini)
Eggplant: 2 (for One-Pot Eggplant and Chickpea Tagine)
Mushrooms: 1 pound (for Spinach and Mushroom Keto Quiche, Mushroom and Wild Rice Pilaf)
Garlic: 2 bulbs (for various recipes)
Onions: 6 (for various recipes)
Beets: 2 (for Beet and Walnut Hummus with Crudités, Ginger and Turmeric Bliss Balls)
Cucumbers: 2 (for Cucumber and Dill Greek Yogurt Dip)
Herbs: Fresh parsley, basil, cilantro, dill (for various recipes)

Grains & Bakery:

Quinoa: 2 cups (for One-Pot Mediterranean Pasta with Olives, Herb-Roasted Chicken with Quinoa Pilaf)
Brown Rice: 1 cup (for Spicy Chickpea and Brown Rice Bowl)
Bulgur Wheat: 1 cup (for Lentil and Bulgur Wheat Salad)
Wild Rice: 1 cup (for Mushroom and Wild Rice Pilaf)
Whole Grain Bread: 1 loaf (for Mini Avocado Toasts with Tomato)
Almond Flour: 1 cup (for Almond Flour Waffles with Cottage Cheese)
Polenta: 1 tube (for Baked Polenta with Marinara and Mushrooms)

Nuts & Seeds:

Walnuts: 1 cup (for Beet and Walnut Hummus with Crudités)
Pumpkin Seeds: 1/2 cup (for Ginger and Turmeric Bliss Balls)
Chia Seeds: 1/2 cup (for various recipes)

Pantry Staples:

Olive Oil: 1 bottle (for various recipes)
Coconut Oil: 1 jar (for various recipes)
Low Carb Sweetener: 1 package (for various recipes)
Soy Sauce: 1 bottle (for One-Pot Mediterranean Pasta with Olives)
Balsamic Vinegar: 1 bottle (for Balsamic Chicken and Roasted Vegetables)
Paprika: 1 jar (for Classic Hummus with Paprika)
Turmeric: 1 jar (for various recipes)
Ground Cinnamon: 1 jar (for Lemon Poppy Seed Porridge)
Salt and Pepper: 1 set (for various recipes)

Miscellaneous:

Cocoa Powder: 1 container (for Ginger and Turmeric Bliss Balls)
Dark Chocolate: 1 bar (for Ginger and Turmeric Bliss Balls)
Vanilla Extract: 1 bottle (for various recipes)

Made in United States
Orlando, FL
19 October 2024

52763908R10046